The Book on Greatness

How to Keep Shining Your Light

Mary Pulles Cavanaugh

Disclaimer: The information in this book is designed to provide helpful information on the subjects discussed. This book is not meant to be used, nor should it be used to diagnose or treat any medical condition or give any medical, financial, legal, psychological or any other kind of professional advice.

© 2016 MARY PULLES CAVANAUGH

ALL RIGHTS RESERVED. NO PART OF THIS WORK MAY BE REPRODUCED OR STORED IN AN INFORMATIONAL RETRIEVAL SYSTEM, WITHOUT THE EXPRESS PERMISSION OF THE PUBLISHER IN WRITING.

ISBN-13: 978-1530700172
ISBN-10: 1530700175

PUBLISHED BY:
10-10-10 PUBLISHING
MARKHAM, ON
CANADA

Contents

Foreword	v
Chapter 1: Introduction	1
Chapter 2: Pre-Conception Through Pre-school	11
Chapter 3: School	23
Chapter 4: Healthcare or Sickcare	37
Chapter 5: Autism AKA Vaccine Induced Brain Injury	55
Chapter 6: Dr./Healers - Who Are They?	75
Chapter 7: My Father's Story	85
Chapter 8: Personal Development	99
Chapter 9: Mother's Pain and Call to Action	109
Acknowledgements	117
About the Author	121
Resources	123

FOREWORD

This book will take you on a journey to discover your inner healing power and your amazing mind. Mary will teach you to gain different healing modalities and by using her methods she will lead you to long-lasting health and greatness.

Most importantly, Mary will provide you with the knowledge so your body's innate ability to heal will remain protected and your brain will continue to grow. Her ongoing journey of 18 years, beginning with the vaccine-induced brain injury of her youngest daughter, the sudden death of her mother-in-law, and her father's very long slow state of chronic neuron-degeneration has opened her eyes and ears to information that is waiting to be shared with you. Many families have had to slowly or very quickly watch loved ones slip away from them. The pain of this kind of death never goes away, and a great void is present. Deep down, you will see the unnaturalness of this and will be haunted by it. It is in this humanness that you will search for answers and truth. May the God-inspired words Mary has penned in this book begin to open your doors of pain and unleash your greatness where the ripple effect of your vibrations will be felt wherever you go.

Raymond Aaron
NY Times Bestselling Author

.

This book is dedicated to all the Allopathic Physicians and Pharmacists who are blindly causing harm under the direction of the CDC, FDA, and Pharmaceutical Companies. It is my prayer you will put your work on pause and discover how the body and brain really work.

Chapter 1
MY BACKGROUND

I am a mom of three daughters who now realizes there are things I would do differently when it comes to my health and my family's health. I was more concerned with the material items my babies needed than what was being done to my body and in turn my growing baby. If only I had spent as much time researching medical procedures as I did what car seat or stroller to buy. You see, back then I was what I like to call a sheeple, I followed the herd. I trusted my midwife. When my midwife told me I needed a rhogam shot during pregnancy I never questioned her. I was told I needed this because I had negative blood and my husband had positive blood. I did not know that the rhogam in 1989 contained 12.5 mcg. of thimerosal, a form of ethyl mercury which is a neurotoxin.

In hindsight I am wondering now why this was only required for my first child? How many things are we being told that are not really true? A family practitioner I know tells me he gets his directives concerning shots from the Center for Disease Control. Do midwives get their directives there too?

I was aware at the time that I wanted a midwife because I was under the impression that I would have more control of my birth and I wanted as natural of a birth as possible. Thankfully I lived in CA where midwives were allowed. My former state, Alabama, 26 years later still do not allow midwives. My husband and I enrolled in Bradley classes to give us all the knowledge so a natural birth could be a reality for us. The Bradley Method is a husband-coached natural childbirth which also emphasizes a well balanced diet of 100 grams of protein daily.

I also made the decision not to use a birthing center because in the case of an emergency I wanted a neonatal intensive care nursery on site. Now looking back at that decision, on the day my 2nd daughter was born I was 10 days late and that day my midwife had stripped my membranes. My water broke around dinner time and there was no time to go to the hospital which gave my husband the privilege of delivering his 2nd daughter!!! We also were not allowed to go to the hospital of our midwife because we were out of the jurisdiction of the ambulance company. So the hospital we were taken to did not even have a neonatal intensive care unit. I should have had more faith in God's design of the birth of a baby. Why did I lose confidence in what is a perfectly natural process?

Twenty six years later I see hospitals marketing their beautiful rooms, water births, and yet I hear horror stories from woman who have a completely different experience than what they have been promised. In fact there is a lawsuit pending in a hospital in Birmingham, AL exactly relating to this.

Looking back now I realize I have three daughters who have been vaccine injured in different ways. I was blessed that they did not receive a low functioning "autism" diagnosis. Their vaccine injury looked like: gastric reflux, severe gastrointestinal pain, inability to go up and down escalators and elevators due to balance/brain issues, developmental delays, struggling cognitively, becoming clumsy, anxiety, inability to sleep, loss of some eye contact, ADD, ADHD diagnosis (2 of the girls), not being able to tie shoes and to this day struggling to ride a bike. This is not OK and is not acceptable. Also, we received an ADD diagnosis in high school having never gotten that diagnosis previously. My youngest daughter suffered from severe meltdowns to the point where both our lives where in jeopardy. She had no control of what was happening to her and many times the meltdown was repeated again. Remember, the younger the child the more vaccines were required on the CDC schedule.

In 2008 my "Autism" journey began, shortly after my youngest daughter received the diagnosis of PDD-NOS. This stands for Pervasive Developmental Disorder None Other Specified. A few months after my daughter received this diagnosis I attended a Defeat Autism Now Conference in my town. It was there that I learned about a study involving monkeys. The monkeys were given the very same vaccine schedule that was recommended by the Center For Disease Control. As a result of this insult the monkeys showed symptoms of Autism. I learned that the mercury in the vaccines was playing a role in this.[1]

2nd Thru 5th grade

Prior to the PDD-NOS diagnosis: my daughter was given the ADHD diagnosis in second grade. My youngest would voice to me often how she hated school. I learned later that her name was a constant

---

[1] Hewitson L, Lopresti BJ, et al. Influence of pediatric vaccines on amygdala growth and opioid ligand binding in rhesus macaque infants: a pilot study. Acta Neurobiol Exp 2010; 70: 147-64.

addition to the daily board work not to mention on the classroom door. There was an ADD/ADHD screening test called the Connor Rating Scale that was in use in the schools at the time. My daughter scored very high on this test and soon afterwards we found ourselves in our pediatrician's office being handed samples of a psychotropic medication for her ADHD within 15 minutes during our appointment. Her school work that I had brought with me was not even given a glance by the "Dr." We were also given a referral to a Developmental Pediatrician who turned out to be another drug pusher.

Given the negative environment at her public school I made the decision to put my daughter in a Charter School. Upon inquiry I learned that tutoring at this school would also be available to her and that was also beginning to look like a necessity. During this time I got familiar with the terms 504 plan and IEP (Individual Educational Plan). Even with the ADHD diagnosis and a letter from the Developmental Pediatrician stating my daughter needed extra time when testing, this request was not granted. I was also unable to obtain a 504 or an IEP despite several attempts. My daughter was an above average student and just for that reason alone she was not considered a candidate. My daughter was also not allowed to be invited on the Honor Roll because of her conduct issues. I had many conversations with the principal about ADHD and how it affects children cognitively and behaviorally but she refused to give any consideration for this disability. Ironically my daughter's best grading period was when I took her out of school on a part time basis so she could perform for 6 weeks at a professional level at our local Repertory Theater.

The practitioners we were seeing during 2nd thru 5th grade included a Psychologist, Psychiatrist, Developmental Pediatrician, and a Sleep specialist. On the last day of school I had a conversation with one of my daughter's teachers and she said to me "Your daughter is not in the classroom." When she said this I knew my daughter was physically in the classroom so she was saying she was not in the classroom cognitively. I made the decision right then and there to obtain a Neuropsychological before we went any further with her schooling. I was going to get to the bottom of this come hell or high water!!!

MIDDLE SCHOOL

I obtained the Neuropsychological the summer before she entered 6th grade. I did this privately and was able to get my insurance company to cover it, which was a miracle. My Neuropsychologist was so angry that my insurance company had kept him on the phone for over an hour he told me that he will never accept any patient with my insurance again!

One of the suggestions that were made by the Neuropsychologist was to take my daughter to an Occupational Therapist. By the time 6th grade started I had armed myself with a private Neuropsychological and an assessment from an Occupational Therapist which gave us a new diagnosis to add called Sensory Processing Disorder. She also received the diagnosis of Hypotonia at this time. The characteristics of Hypotonia are low muscle tone and low muscle strength. I now understood why she could not hold her pencil properly and why she always craved deep pressure in the form of lots of hugs.

Prior to the meeting at the middle school to determine my daughters IEP eligibility I had also discovered a website called wrightslaw.com. The owner of the website was the attorney that actually fights the special education cases that go before the Supreme Court. This website gave me just what I needed to arm myself with the parts of the law that pertained to my daughter's disability. I also learned somewhere along the way to get a picture of my daughter in a picture frame and put it in middle of the conference table. I also hired a special education advocate, not necessarily because I did not have the knowledge that she had but because I was so close to the situation it was imperative that I keep my emotions in check. I found myself quoting the law instead of the advocate and because of this cited law I was able to keep my daughter out of a self-contained classroom that was located offsite. Now armed with an IEP my daughter was able to qualify for a McKay Scholarship that my state offered. This is a tuition stipend that can be used for any approved private school.

The private school that I chose was a Montessori School and for the first year everything flowed quite nicely. Thankfully the classes were small and the principal was also a friend of mine. Hands-on learning proved to be a good match for my daughter. She also had the opportunity to learn an instrument. Music came very naturally to her. Unfortunately the practicing did not and this hobby was short lived. She also participated in the school swim team albeit at times begrudgingly. At times the outside temperature was cool or it was raining and this was not her idea of fun. She was also at the beginning of puberty and a very volatile period in our relationship. On a positive note singing was her passion. She had perfect pitch and could always tell if something was out of tune instinctively. She also could match a singer's voice to the notes that she could sing. The right side of her brain was definitely operating at a higher level.

So fast forward to 7th grade and things were getting even more volatile. At that time we began seeing a specialist in Vision Processing who happened to be an hour away. During this time it was very difficult to get my daughter in the car let alone out of the car. Going to appointments became a real challenge even though we were beginning to work on integrating her left and right side of her brain and body. For example, she now had the ability to tell right from left. It was at this time that the Eye Specialist suggested to me that my daughter be tested for heavy metal toxicity through a hair analysis test. I took the kit to the hair dresser and we followed instructions and I sent it off. The heavy metal toxicity test revealed that my daughter was off the charts in copper, magnesium, and very high in manganese. After I saw these test results I took them to our Holistic Pediatrician that we had just began seeing. When I showed him the results he told me my daughter should never be vaccinated again. He also told me that he was currently shadowing a Defeat Autism Now doctor in Tampa and he will refer me there. I pretty much told him that I no longer wanted to hear about "autism" and I was interested in treating the heavy metal toxicity. Thankfully he totally got it!

Within 2 weeks my husband and I with our daughter found ourselves driving to Tampa to see this Biomedical Doctor. I was so thankful that my daughter cooperated on that day. We were immediately given a prescription to order from a compounding pharmacy for a glutathione cream that you put on the skin with the instructions to start epsom salt baths immediately for the next week; two cups, twenty minutes a night. Yes we had to put a TV in the bathroom but we were willing to do whatever it took.

Just with that protocol alone we witnessed a calming that came over my daughter. The PTSD (Post Traumatic Stress Disorder) state that I was always in was starting to see some daylight. Just that treatment alone made a difference for us. We found the major meltdowns going down dramatically once we started the glutathione protocol.

An Organic Acid profile test was also ordered that we performed at home. This test indicated she was low in glutathione. I soon learned that if you are low in glutathione your body's detoxification pathways are compromised. Glutathione is your body's major antioxidant. It is also your body's major anti-inflammatory of which "autism" is a very inflammatory condition of the brain and body. It also regulates ATP which is related to our energy. After finding out the role of glutathione in the body and my daughter's lack of it I began to get an understanding of why her behavior was so difficult. In my independent studies I learned that behavior is how a child sees, how a child hears, and how a child feels. Things were starting to become a little clearer to me. The research that I began in earnest when my daughter hit puberty was beginning to pay off.

The social media site Linked In was one of my teachers. I became a voracious reader. I had Amazon on speed dial. I became an attendee of many webinars and teleconferences. My attendance at Autismone in Chicago every year was a no brainer. Pubmed.gov became my best friend and helped me win my case with Aetna and I was able to get our out of network Biomedical Dr. covered. Not only did they pay for the visits I was also able to get coverage for the labs and supplements that were ordered. At the end of this chapter is the compiled research that won my case!

Purpose

My purpose in writing this book is to empower you to the greatness that is inside you. Did you know that your wonderfully made body is always making new cells? The part of our eye called cones, which is responsible for color and how the eye functions, is shed every 2-3 days. So is the inner side of our stomach. Every six weeks we get new skin and every eight weeks a new liver!!! This is mind blowing to me but so exciting to know. We really are fearfully and wonderfully made!!!

I also feel like it is important to be given the opportunity to use all kinds of venues to educate you with this information so you can avoid my pain in many of my family's medical conditions. I would also like to live in the abundance that our maker promises all of us so I can become a woman of influence and right the wrongs that have been committed by big pharma, the CDC and the physicians who practice the allopathic model.

What I Will Cover

My perspective is rather unique in that I come from the background of being a Child Protective Service Worker for three years and a Substitute Teacher for 10 years and counting. I will also be covering, in the following chapters, healthcare or what I like to call sickcare. I will also talk about what I learned as I watched my father's health very slowly decline. I will also talk about what I experienced in the hospital with my late mother-in-law.

This journey has led me to fall in love with the brain. I also discovered healing powers that I did not know we had. I will explain the Dr./Healers/Practitioners that are out there that embrace wellness. I will cover your inner healing power and all the healing modalities that are available to enhance that. I also cannot leave out how this journey has led me to network marketing and what I feel is the most important benefit that I was introduced to which is personal development. To have the knowledge that there is a hospital in China which uses no drugs to treat their patients. In lieu of drugs they use chants. Gregg Braden is the visionary whom I heard that from. So that is a snippet of what is waiting in chapter eight. The last chapter gives examples of mother's pain and I ask for a call to action. I do not think anyone wants to lose their medical freedom and it is my hope and prayer that in the end you will choose to join me in this very important cause.

Chapter 2
PRE-CONCEPTION THROUGH PRESCHOOL

Detox and Diet

In this Chapter I will teach you the pitfalls to avoid so you and your children can stay in wellness. I would have liked to have had on my radar the knowledge of whether my body had the ability to detox. To find out a kit can be ordered from www.23andme.com. I have seen commercials for these kits on ESPN! It is becoming more and more mainstream to seek knowledge about the genetic make up of your family. Anyone with the MTHFR gene should never vaccinate because their detoxification pathways are compromised. MTHFR stands for methyl-tetrahydrofolate. This is the enzyme that is responsible for the methylation (detox) of every cell in your body. I highly recommend that every parent have their family screened for this. So there you have it vaccines are not one size fits all!!!

Another area to look at before conception is diet. Your diet should be as clean as possible. By clean I mean no preservatives, artificial flavors, enriched wheat, hydrogenated or fractionated oils, additives, dyes, monosodium glutamate, sugar, acesulfame-K, sucralose, aspartame, high fructose corn syrup, gluten (glyphosate), propyl gallate, potassium benzoate, sodium benzoate, potassium sorbate, soy lecithin, sodium chloride, polysorbate 80, soy, corn, canola oil, casein, and GMO'S (genetically modified organisms). If the ingredient list is more than 5, buyer beware. If you cannot pronounce the ingredient that is another red flag. Our food needs to come from its natural source. We need to go back to a hunter and gatherer diet. A lot of our food is being tampered with for profit and we need to remain as vigilant as possible.

It is also important to look at the ingredients of beauty products and cleaning products. Anything you put on your skin goes into your bloodstream in about 26 seconds. Think of your skin as a protective cover with many layers underneath including dead cells. The other layers are composed of living cells which respond to irritants when they get through. When these irritants are toxic, problems can occur. The lymphatic system is a network of tissues and organs which help rid the body of toxins, keep the bodily fluids in balance, and fight infections. It carries the lymph which is made up of water, protein molecules, salts, glucose, and other substances. Lymph is continuously leaking out of the tiny blood capillaries into the body tissues. If this excess fluid is not drained the tissues of the body will become swollen.[2] The four stages of inflammation are redness, pain, heat, and swelling. When you have an understanding of how this system works it is easy to see how toxicity can occur. This skin toxicity can lead to blood poisoning. The symptoms of blood poisoning include chills, moderate or high fever, rapid breathing, an increased heart rate or palpitations, and paleness.[3] Interesting to note is all these side effects have also been seen after vaccinations have been administered. I

---

[2] "Blood Poisoning." Healthline. Web. 20 Mar. 2016.
[3] "Spleen and Lymphatic System." Kidshealth - the Web's Most Visited Site about Children's Health. The Nemours Foundation. Web. 20 Mar 2016.

believe vaccinations are poisoning the blood and compromising the lymphatic system.

In 2004 there was a study done by the Environmental Working Group who commissioned five laboratories to examine the umbilical cord blood of 10 babies of African-American, Hispanic and Asian heritage. There were 232 chemicals found in each newborn! The most alarming chemical present is BPA (bisphenol A) which is commonly found in plastic. This contaminant mimics estrogen and has been shown to cause developmental problems and precancerous growth in animals. This finding in this study alone stresses the importance of detoxing prior to conception so as to keep your toxicity to a minimum.

I also would have liked to have more of an understanding of folic acid. This was something I was told to take by my midwife for all three pregnancies and I never questioned it. I have since learned that everyone cannot take folic acid and if you are a candidate for the MTHFR this would be contraindicated.

Choosing a Dr. and Birth Setting

During my pregnancy I spent some time researching a pediatrician. I even set up an interview with him. Unfortunately for me I never questioned any medical intervention so it was not necessary in my mind to second guess a doctor. After all he went to Medical School and I did not.

After seeing the harm that came to my children I now have a completely different mindset when it comes to pediatricians. In fact I have come to the understanding that the Pediatric Specialty's sole purpose is to monitor vaccine immunizations. I also have awoken to the fact that what is learned in Medical School is dictated by Big Pharma. In fact many doctors who teach at Medical Schools are very generously compensated by Big Pharma. If I were to have a baby today I would not even consider a pediatrician unless they understood the ineffectiveness and danger of vaccines today and practiced accordingly. It is not necessary to choose a pediatrician as your baby's doctor. A vaccine friendly doctor can also be a family practitioner, chiropractor, naturopath, osteopath or homeopath. It is so important to choose a practitioner that will offer the freedom of choice when it comes to any medical intervention including vaccines.

Another decision to make is where to have your baby. If I were to choose now it would either be at a birthing center or at my home. These two choices have less probability of being bullied into procedures I am not willing to participate in. There have been cases of births in hospitals where the baby was vaccinated against the parents will. There have also been cases where the baby was ready to come and for reasons of practitioner convenience the birth was delayed. Also mothers were not allowed to birth in the position that they felt most comfortable, natural, and where gravity was being used. This was one of the reasons I chose a Midwife even in the 80's and 90's because they were more in the mindset of allowing the birth to happen naturally with as little intervention as necessary.

Consent Form and Procedures After Birth

There are 3 routine medical interventions that are performed upon the arrival of the baby. They are as follows: 1) Vitamin K which is administered as an intramuscular injection to prevent a RARE newborn condition called hemolytic disease where the babies blood is unable to clot resulting in a possible hemorrhage. This occurs in 1 in 10,000 births and bleeding can occur up to 12 weeks. If I would choose this procedure I would want to make sure the Vitamin K was clean (ie was preservative free). 2) Eye ointment which prevents neonatal infection from STD's. If the mother does not have an STD this procedure is completely unnecessary and can cause the intestinal flora to be compromised and cause a chemical irritation, or interfere with baby's initial eye contact and bonding with mom. 3) Hepatitis B is given to all babies even though the disease is only transmitted through needles and sex. The concern about the Hepatitis B vaccine is it can also lead to compromised reflexes.[4] This can be observed when the baby is born taking right to the breast and after the Hepatitis B vaccine is administered nursing becomes problematic. Another warning about the Hepatitis vaccine is that this vaccine is also being given to preemies but in the same dosage as a full term baby. The weight of a premature baby is less than a full term baby. It has also been my experience when any drug is administered to children weight is always a criterion when deciding the dosage. I have been told that the nurses know to get the crash carts out in the neonatal intensive care unit when the Hepatitis

---

[4] Hewitson L, Houser LA, et al. Delayed acquisition of neonatal reflexes in newborn primates receiving a thimerosal-containing hepatitis B vaccine: influence of gestational age and birth weight. J Toxicol Environ Health A, 2010; 73(19): 1298-1313.

B vaccine is being given to this population because of the compromised breathing that ensues.

Also upon arrival at the hospital a consent form is required. This is something to be taken very seriously. Once a consent form is signed all control is lost. In fact you may want to consider having your attorney go over this consent form prior to your hospital admission. The problem occurs when consent to procedures is not agreed upon by the patient.

Child Abuse Pediatric Specialist

Something that is not widely known is there is now a specialty in medicine called Child Abuse Pediatric. These specialists are liaisons for Child Protective Services and are who the ER Doctors rely on should they run into non compliance with a parent or guardian with a procedure that they deem necessary. Medical kidnapping is alive and well in this country! Mothers have had their newborn infants taken away because of noncompliance of procedures that they believe could be harmful to their child. This is a topic that particularly hits home for me because I am a former Child Protective Service Worker. My role used to be protecting children. Now I find myself protecting innocent caring parents or guardians from Social Workers in my former field of Child Protective Services.

My last note of caution to be aware of is that in some states hospitals are now requiring family members and friends, prior to being allowed to see the baby in the hospital, to be vaccinated. This may be another consideration in your decision as to where to birth your baby.

Back Home

When I brought my older daughter home from the hospital I remember she would not stop pooping. Just as soon as I had cleaned her up she had another bowel movement. In the end I had eight dirty diapers lined up. In the middle of this I found it rather alarming and called the hospital in a panic about it asking them what to do. The answer they gave me was she was probably cleaning herself out. I have always wondered whether there was something else going on and I would actually like to explore this further because I am not sure I should be satisfied with that explanation.

When I brought my middle fully vaccinated daughter home from the hospital she actually screamed from 12 am to 2 am every night for the first 2 months. I remember how helpless I felt when I had to leave my room and go into the nursery where I had set up a chair that opened up and I would lay down on my back with my daughter tummy to tummy until I could calm her two hours later. When I called my pediatrician about getting some understanding of why this was happening I was told she had colic and I was given colic drops which gave her no relief. I now know she was having gastrointestinal issues and despite her pain vaccinations continued on schedule. When babies cry constantly and consistently for that long of a period they are in pain!!! This is not normal!!!

Fast forward to now about a quarter of a century later, the problems I see moms having with their babies include gastric reflux, problems sleeping, constant crying, breastfeeding issues, seizures, developmental delays, skin problems like various rashes and eczema, no eye contact and tongue ties. Tongue ties seem to be very common because a facebook group about tongue tie issues has over 35,000 members!!! This was rarely talked about in my play groups.

The skin problems occur because it is the secondary way the body detoxes, if it cannot detox through the primary way. (kidneys and the liver). I am also very alarmed in seeing babies being given the same medication for gastric reflux as adults. On a personal note my oldest daughter as an infant also suffered from projectile vomiting and reflux. She was my baby which required a diaper on my shoulder at all times for the clean up. My pediatrician at the time never gave me an indication that this was not normal and thankfully treatment back then did not include the proton pump inhibitors of today.

"Well Baby" Checkups

Let's talk about the history of Well Baby checkups which I find the name itself to be the exact opposite of what it suggests. The Well Baby checkup schedule is made up according to the recommended vaccines set by age according to the Center For Disease Control. Everyone is treated the same. The inability to methylate (detox) is not even a consideration.

In regard to the number of vaccines that are being given here is a little background. In 1983 they gave a total of 24 doses from birth through age 18. There were 11 vaccines in total. Now this year that number has escalated to 56 vaccines totaling 74 doses. How can this happen? Well there is no longer any skin in the game for the vaccine manufacturers thanks to the Childhood Vaccine Injury Act passed by Congress in 1986. This act frees them from all liability resulting from vaccine injury or death.

When I was raising my daughters in late 80's thru mid 90's my Well Baby check up consisted of taking the height, weight, and head circumference of the baby. Also recommended shots were administered but never amounted to more than two. I now know two shots were too many for my youngest daughter but at the time I was unaware of the impending danger. I never questioned why they would measure the head circumference. I now believe it was to check for brain development abnormalities although most practitioners would never admit that.

I do recall at my youngest daughter's 2 year old Well Baby checkup I was asked to sign my initials by the vaccines that were being administered. That was the first time that I had been asked to do this. I did ask why this was now required and was told this was just something they were doing now with no additional explanation as to why. If you go to most pediatricians today there is a form to read and sign if you do not agree to vaccinate. This is their way of scaring you into deciding to vaccinate. Do not fall for this. Listen to your mommy gut and have all your research completed prior to your Well Baby visit. Personally, until they green the vaccines and they are held liable should injury or death occur I would not engage in this health intervention.

If you find yourself being bullied into getting vaccines I would highly recommend taking before and after pictures. In some children characteristic traits resembling a stroke can appear on one side of the face very soon after having received the vaccine. Changes in the eyes can also occur. The late Dr. Andrew Moulden has done amazing work on this topic. In the case of a death or injury please make sure you and your "doctor" file a report with VAERS. It is common knowledge that many of these reports do not get filed either by the pediatrician or by the attending doctor in the Emergency Room. This stands for the Vaccine Adverse Event Reporting System. There are 3 years to file a claim with the Vaccine Injury Claims Court. This Court has already given out over 3.5 billion dollars in settlements. In my case we missed that window because we failed to recognize the developmental delays in time. This is very common because sometimes it takes a while for all these vaccine assaults to surface to where you begin to understand that something has gone horribly wrong and you begin to dig deeper.

Developmental Delays Your Doctor May Not Reveal

Here are some symptoms I missed in my youngest daughter: coming down with temporary asthma, eczema, refusing to ride elevators and escalators, always wanting hugs, very high fever the night of the vaccines being administered, difficulty changing activities, always wanting to be carried at an inappropriate age, could not tie shoes or ride a bike till 2nd grade, very sensitive when brushing her hair or grazing her skin, always tired, would always lay down and sleep during church, and could not talk to me when the radio was on in the car. Little did I know she had Sensory Processing Disorder, Visual Processing Disorder, Auditory Processing Disorder, and difficulty with balance. Not once did her pediatrician suggest something may be wrong and continued to assault her with vaccines through Kindergarten. How do all these diagnoses affect school performance? My next chapter will be painting that picture.

Chapter 3
SCHOOL

Immunization Exemptions

I am a mother of a child with a language based learning disability that came from an acquired traumatic brain injury. I am also in my tenth year of substitute teaching. This gives me the background I need to talk about a passion of mine which is finding out more about what has happened to the school children and their learning environment.

The first thing you will be asked to give the school upon entering school is your child's immunization form. Many schools state this is required which could not be further from the truth. There are three kinds of exemption forms that can be obtained depending on your state mandate. States differ in regard to what exemptions they will accept. The three kinds are Philosophical, Religious, and Medical. It is unconscionable that schools are lying to the parents about this when there is a large part of the population that is being harmed. In fact ironically what is needed to excel in school, which is a great brain, is being compromised by this medical procedure. Many children in the United States are continuing to be compromised both cognitively in the classroom as well as in their athletic ability that is needed to excel in sports.

My personal experience took place in the state of Florida in my child's middle school years. This was when I made the decision that my child was not going to get anymore vaccines after I made the connection between what the ingredients in the vaccine do to the body and brain. By this time we had the PDD-NOS (Pervasive Developmental Disorder None Other Specified) diagnosis. I first called a local DAN (Defeat Autism Now) Doctor to see if she could give me a medical exemption since I had the "autism" diagnosis. I was told I had to go to my local health department. I decided to call them first. I explained my child's diagnosis and they just told me I just needed to come in and they would give me the form I needed. The year was 2007. I was shocked that they did not require any documentation to verify what I had just told them and I also did not need to bring my child. I walked in and there were two lists on a table to sign. One list was for parents who knew that vaccines were not required if you get an exemption and another list for parents who just assumed vaccines were mandated. When they called me back to sign the medical exemption they said "Well you know Mrs. Cavanaugh, your child will not be able to attend school should these diseases appear at the school. She may return only after these diseases have been eradicated." I was dumbfounded at the obvious absurdity of what she just told me but my mission was accomplished. I have also been made fully aware by a very smart naturopath in a company I was in at the time that all D I S E A S E is inflammation, acidosis, oxidative stress, and dehydration.

Fast forward two years later when my daughter was changing schools again. This time I walked in and asked for a Medical exemption. The lady said "You mean you want a religious exemption?" I said "No

I want a medical exemption." She said again "Do you want a religious exemption?" By this time I was getting annoyed and I looked at her and said "Just give me whatever I need." I have come to realize that NOW medical exemptions can only come from a certain type of "Doctor" The same ones that administer the vaccines....fancy that!

As an original member of the Autism Mitochondrial Task Force which originated in Boston in the late 2000's, I learned that a doctor who has been involved in the mitochondrial disease since its inception has the belief that oxidative stress is the culprit that is deleting the mitochondrial DNA that we continue to see today. What is causing oxidative stress? Oxidative stress is the production of free radicals. What are free radicals? Free radicals are unpaired electrons. Vaccines cause a lot of free radical damage which means these unpaired electrons go all around the cell damaging everything in their path. Where is this free radical damage coming from?

What Is In Vaccines

Have you ever looked at what is in the vaccines? I find it incredible that the "Doctors" who administer these shots have absolutely no idea what they contain. I guess no news is bad news right? Unfortunately there is a lot of bad news. Here are some of the ingredients in the vaccines: monosodium glutamate, anti-freeze, formaldehyde, aluminum, glycerin, lead, cadmium, sulfates, yeast, proteins, antibiotics, acetone, neomycin, streptomycin, mercury, monkey kidney, dog kidney, chick embryo, chicken egg, duck egg, calf serum, aborted fetal cell tissue, pig blood, horse blood, sheep blood, rabbit brain, guinea pig, cow heart, animal viruses, insect cells, silk worm

DNA, etc......!!! A card with these vaccine ingredients on it can be obtained free of charge at vacinfo.org.

Classroom Environment

Let us now go inside the classroom and look at how the lighting, sound, and electromagnetic field pollution can hinder a child's learning. Ever since my daughter was diagnosed with a Sensory Processing Disorder and I learned what it is I became very conscious of what lighting, sound, and the electromagnetic field is doing to her body and how her behavior was being affected.

Going back to my own experience with florescent lights I remember in my 8th grade typing class sitting at my desk with my eyes just tearing up. Florescent lights are commonly used in schools. During my independent study of "Autism" I became very intrigued with how "Autism" has compromised the frequency of the cells. Light in particular can raise the frequency of the cells. We know light can affect how you feel. We see this often in countries that have less daylight like the United Kingdom. People there can suffer from SAD also called Seasonal Affective Disorder. Over the years I was also made aware of the change in the light bulbs that are now available to buy. We were now being told that these energy efficient bulbs will save us money. These are the same ones that contain mercury and a hazmat crew is needed if one should accidentally be dropped. At first I bought several for our home until I realized the light is not nearly as bright as the natural light and furthermore I did not feel well around it. So as I studied this I found out architect Randall Fielding cited research demonstrating that naturally lit classrooms increased verbal scores by

22 percent and math scores by 20 percent. The research also showed that lighting that was too dim lead to learning difficulties which affected how the brain focused and the visual clarity of the eyes. It eventually lowered the psychological well being of the student. To the contrary, florescent lighting contributed to off task and worsening behavior. This academic achievement study in children took place in 1999 at the University of Georgia.

With so many children receiving the diagnosis of Sensory Processing Disorder the level of sound in the classroom can play a role in classroom performance and behavior. Around the year 2000 I recall walking into classrooms and observing tennis balls on the ends of the legs from the desk chairs. I also recall having been asked to buy tennis balls one year just for that purpose. To my knowledge this was not a concern in previous years. I do think many of us have yet to grasp how the frequency of sound can affect behavior or affect how the body feels. The children who are most affected by the electromagnetic field (EMF) are children on the Autism spectrum, children with ADHD (Attention Deficit Hyperactivity Disorder), and children with ADD (Attention Deficit Disorder). During my health journey I was invited to attend a whole day of presentations at this very well known local Integrative Doctor's office. Part of the day included getting screened by his chiropractor for susceptibility to the EMF. It turned out that this did not appear to be a problem for me. This susceptibility to the EMF is as individualized as vaccine harm. The healthier your cells are the less susceptible you will be.

There are two experiences that I have had that have made an impact in my knowledge in this area. There was a friend I met through a company that we were both in at the time that was actually poisoned by the electrical power lines in her backyard. It turned out the electrical power had been increased and the neighborhood had not been given any notice ahead of time. Many conversations with my friend followed and I learned how many of her EMF sickness symptoms mimicked what we see in "Autism" aka vaccine induced injury. I began to understand why my daughter made these weird high pitched humming noises when she got near the refrigerator. She also would repeat this noise when we drove past the Wi-Fi tower on the campus of her high school. I also learned that just as in "Autism" the blood brain barrier becomes compromised with EMF poisoning. My friend has also written a book about her story which can be found here at backyardsecretexposed.com

The second experience involved a lady I met who was filling in at a vintage shop that I stopped in to look for a costume for my daughter's musical. A conversation ensued and I mentioned the book I had co-authored with the Thinking Moms and then she proceeded to tell me about her previous work involving microprocessors. She was extremely interested in my story. I then had a light bulb moment when she told me she was sick and I asked her if the heavy metals made her more susceptible to EMF poisoning and she replied in the affirmative. WOW!!! She proceeded to tell me everyone in the plant had gotten sick and a lawsuit was filed and they won. The building was taken down and she said even the footprint is gone. WOW! After that conversation I became even more convinced that I needed to avoid heavy metals at all cost.

So the next question we need to ask ourselves is what has increased the EMF in school? I know that in the middle schools I substitute at, two thirds of the students in my classes have cell phones. There could be cellular antennas radiating to the school from nearby buildings or cellular antennas radiating from the school building to another building with glass windows that reflects the radio frequency back to you. At schools we now see cellular towers or antennas on campus or adjacent to campus. This may include hidden or stealth cell site installations built on the roof or inside chimney or church steeples. We now have wireless networks, wireless access points, wireless laptop, plus wireless overhead projectors and whiteboards that are used for interactive learning in the classroom. Ironically some teachers will wear FM transmitters for hearing impaired students that emit excessively high radio frequency exposures or chronic exposures. If this is the case a desk placement is preferred.

Cursive Writing, Telling Time, and Math Struggles

Another change that is happening in many schools today is the disappearance of cursive writing. I myself find this stunning. When you write in cursive you develop your muscle control and your eye hand coordination. Eye hand coordination is also key to being a success in sports. When you write in script your motion is fluid and this enhances your hand eye coordination, develops fine motor skills, and promotes reading, writing, and cognition skills. Writing in cursive is also faster than printing. When you print you pick up your writing implement after printing each letter. Interestingly enough since cursive writing is no longer being taught in many schools, occupational therapy costs have risen. When I see a paper from a child that has sloppy handwriting my first thought is this is related to fine motor control. Writing in cursive also stimulates the brain in a variety of ways. The repetition that is involved in writing in script fashion helps ingrain skills and information in the brain. Just the movement involving the hand and also the eyes following the script writing is a wonderful brain exercise. You have to wonder if there is an ulterior motive here. The children who do not acquire this skill will not have the ability to interpret historical documents of which many are written in cursive. They will also be unable to read their ancestors letters and journals. I also wonder if teacher laziness is playing a part or have the teachers become just overwhelmed because of the multiple exceptionalities they have to deal with in their classroom setting.

Many diagnoses have sprung up since I was in elementary school. Have you ever heard of dyscalculia? This is a disability that was discovered in 1974 by Dr. Ladislav Rose. This learning disability relates to approximating time and can also include a speech or language delay. Speaking of time, many kids these days cannot tell time on an analog clock. The ability to tell time on a clock involves visual spatial memory. This kind of memory is needed for success in Math. It is also needed later on to drive because this involves estimating speed and distance. Two more skills that lead to success in math are memory and processing. The inability to tell time leads to more struggles later in fractions, equations, conversions and more.

Vision Processing Disorder

I never realized how involved our visual system is when performing math until I attended an Autismone Conference in 2008.

This conference is held every year in Chicago and is the most innovative conference in regard to healing the body and the brain. I will never forget the optometrist that presented there. She said the children who struggle in Math, of which there are many on the Autism spectrum, should never have more than 5 problems on a page. The more I thought about it the more this made a lot of sense to me. So often when you work on problems that involve several steps you are working in a very small space. If you have more than 5 problems on a page everything looks very close together visually. If you have tracking problems you could very easily lose track of which problem you are working on.

Tracking problems are related to a visual processing disorder which also includes how the eye teams and focuses. This also has everything to do with reading comprehension. The public schools solution for this is to put all these children in intensive reading programs. A visual processing disorder involves a problem with how the eye functions physically. This problem creates great difficulty reading because your eyes become very tired and can also tear up from working so hard. Falling asleep can also be a consequence of this. It is stunning to me that the schools have not addressed this problem in regard to offering screenings at the elementary school level. This could be life changing for so many kids if they and their parents were given the knowledge they have this problem and then their parents can have them treated accordingly. I also was made aware that being tested using a scantron could lead to a roadblock with these kids. There was a case where a girl took the SAT test and she filled in the b bubble instead of the c bubble and her disorder caused her to be one off on every answer on her test. Can you imagine how that affected her score? Can you also imagine how this affected where she went to college or if she went to college? When I looked into treating my daughter for this because her Neuropsychological indicated this weakness, I found out there were only four eye doctors in town with this specialty. I found it stunning that the other eye doctors do not even attempt to do an initial screening and then refer on. I believe it is because the therapy for this disorder is not covered by insurance and it is not in the doctor's financial benefit to pursue this. If I was an eye doctor I could not in good conscience practice like this. I would screen for this at a minimum especially if I found out the child was struggling in school. The website to find a provider is covd.org.

I cannot end this topic without stressing how important vision processing is to driving. Now there are some parts of the country where you can get along fine without driving but unless you live in a big city the inability to drive will limit you. I am seeing more and more young people struggling with this basic skill. There are now communities being built with support systems for high functioning young adults on the Autism spectrum who do not want to live at home. Ninety five percent of the residents in these communities do not drive! Is this going to be the norm? I hope not. It is my desire that we discontinue the practices of what is causing this disorder. The vaccines in my mind are highly suspect.

Recess and Physical Education

Did the schools idea of eliminating recess coincide with the implementation of standardized recess and why? Is this about giving teachers more time to teach or is this about getting a better rank or higher scores on standardized tests? Is the discipline, bad manners, and emotional distress that we see in the classrooms today taking teaching time away? Given the fact that many of the children need to move in order for their brains to work, taking recess away borders on cruelty. Recess is about playing. When children play they get the opportunity to express themselves and use their imagination. This is also their time to explore, develop their confidence, practice skills, connect with friends and learn about social survival. Believe it or not this kind of playground education also assists them in how they learn inside the classroom. Many of the skills such as thinking, planning, using trial and error, working through challenges, communicating, expressing frustration, and sharing ideas is exactly what they need to survive inside the classroom too. I cannot help observe the irony in the movement of raising academic standards when the brains of children through medical intervention are being harmed. This harm is causing cognitive delays and an inability to upgrade their academic achievement. I would also urge teachers not to use Physical Education or recess as a punishment. The kids who struggle need movement in order to get their brain to work. I believe writing many sentences in cursive relating to the behavior they are struggling with would be more beneficial to them. This is a great brain exercise and was used successfully as a deterrent in my day.

The kids who struggle in Physical Education are most likely compromised in hand eye coordination. I recently witnessed something that occurs almost daily in PE classes. This concerns the practice of having students pick their classmates for their team sport that they will be playing for the day. Watching this brought back painful memories for me as I was always the last one picked due to my inability to catch a ball because of my vision processing disorder. It is most important that the choosing of teams be done as rapidly as possible because of the emotional pain that comes into play. All you have to do is see the looks of fright, defeat, and failure on the students faces to know this ritual needs to be completed quickly. Because the number of kids who struggle in sports have increased in class I would like to see more emphasis in building the skills needed to improve the hand eye coordination. It is also important to offer a variety of sports so everyone can participate and be successful in their sports performance. For the kids who struggle academically and also athletically the arts become their lifeline. For some this is how they find their purpose in life and their passion. It is for this reason that theater, music, and art should NEVER be on the chopping block. The arts may be the ONLY avenue that these cognitively delayed kids have to excel.

I would also like to talk about troubled kids for a moment. Teachers see these kids in the schools every day. What is going on with them? Many are exhausted when they get up. They barely eat breakfast. They sit alone wearing their headphones on the bus. Many cannot even ride the bus because of the loud stimuli. They lose or forget their assignments and cannot keep up with the work in class. They also cannot keep up with many of their classmate's conversation. They are laughed at by their classmates and admonished by their teachers daily. Their school day ends and they try to do their homework which quickly becomes an impossibility. As a result their parents are also frustrated with them. The next day what I just described gets repeated. Is there any wonder why these kids have anger issues or hate school?

Boys and Puberty

Now let us talk about the boys who the "Doctors" have told us are behind in maturity when compared to girls. Are they really? What do we know? We know mercury is used in some of the vaccines that the boys get. The destructive power of mercury enhances testosterone. Research shows that people with "Autism" have lower levels of glutathione. Testosterone actually blocks the ability of the body to make glutathione. Mercury binds to glutathione thus inactivating whatever glutathione the body may already have. At the same time mercury is raising the testosterone levels it is dramatically lowering the glutathione levels which is the bodies major way to detoxify.

It is interesting to note that in the past 40 years in the United States the age of puberty in girls has dropped 1-2 years. However in the Scandinavian countries, which demanded thimerasal-free vaccines in 1991, there has been no drop in the age of puberty. As a substitute teacher of 10 years, I have observed the change in students in all grades either appearing a lot younger than their age or a lot older than their age. There are kids that are in middle school that look like they could be in third grade and then there are other kids that look like they could be in high school or even college.

School of the Future

If I were to come up with a model of the School of the Future what would it look like? There would be no required vaccines and this would be clearly stated on all correspondence. All lighting would be as close to natural light as possible. All testing would be chosen on an individual basis depending on the strengths of the student. For example my daughter excels when she is tested orally. Teaching to the test would be over and creative teaching would be encouraged. Movement and music would be accepted in the learning process. All children would have access to earphones. Personal Development and Leadership would be required subjects in Middle School and High School. I would like to see a program like lifekinetikusa.com become a required class for all the kids who struggle cognitively in the classroom. Lifekinetik trains the brain using movement which involves crossing the midline. Hands on learning should be emphasized and encouraged whenever possible. All elementary children who struggle in reading will be screened for a vision processing disorder. Also hand sanitizers would be banned from all classrooms unless they are organic in nature. The school would be grounded properly to keep the electromagnetic field pollution at a minimum. Music, Art, and Dance classes would be available in all grades. The library would become the most popular place to go. The food would come from its natural source and there would be a garden on the property. History would be taught in its entirety.

I think some of the ideas in my school of the future are not too far off in reality. There are some private schools that are modeling some of this now. Children are all brilliant and are born learners. They deserve to spend their days in school with a smile on their face. Teachers are also worthy of going home energized instead of in the exhaustive state of today.

CHAPTER 4
HEALTHCARE AND SICKCARE

Medical School and Big Pharma

What is going on in Medical School? Does the wooing start at the undergraduate level? What personality are the Medical Schools looking for? How much influence do pharmaceutical companies have both in the pre-med programs and in Medical School? What is the history of the God complex that is so evident in this field today? What are they leaving out when it comes to inner healing? These are some of the questions I hope to answer.

Let's get started. I cannot talk about these topics without talking about Medical School and Big Pharma. It is my understanding the wooing from pharmaceutical companies does begin with the pre-med students in undergraduate school. I have heard it is not uncommon for pre-med students to have their lunch paid for by a drug company.

I would love to have the opportunity to sit it on a Medical School interview. I am quite certain that they look for a personality that they can mold, shape, and brainwash to their thinking. I find there is very little information out there in regard to this application process.

I have learned during the first two years of Medical School there is absolutely no contact with sales representatives in both the drug and procedure industry in Big Pharma. This all changes in year 3. These sales reps have even been known to hang around the operating room. The hierarchy in medicine is almost indistinguishable in the operating room setting. What I mean by that is everyone in this setting is wearing scrubs and would look the same to an outsider. The sales rep would have no idea who was a doctor, nurse, or medical student.

To find out how Big Pharma operates I find former Pharmaceutical Sales Representatives in the industry are an excellent resource. There are several ways Big Pharma uses to get their products out to the market and to the appropriate medical specialists and practitioners. They do this by giving drug samples to the doctors. They also use educational and non-educational programming. The sales reps also will leave behind advertising specialty items which we always see during our visits in the form of pens, notepads, clips etc. The most popular way is enjoying free champagne, brunches, happy hours, and various event tickets. The money these reps spend on marketing is infinite and when this money is gone there is always more. I would be very leery of doctors with all these drug specialty items around or if I spotted a rep in the waiting room at an appointment. If you would like to see how much money your doctor is being paid by Big Pharma you can look it up at the following website: openpayments.cms.gov At times you may find this website inaccessible.

Allopathic Medicine

Three areas that are very interwoven in allopathic medicine are insurance, drugs, and procedures. I wonder if the tests that insurance companies agree to cover have a direct link to certain drug treatment?

I also know that doctors who practice outside the box of allopathic medicine do not accept insurance. The reason for this is because the tests they perform on their patients the insurance will not cover. What are the criteria the insurance companies use to determine the coverage of a drug or procedure? After some research I discovered they use Medicare as their model. Unfortunately for the patient Medicare has a history of not approving anything that is new to the market. How have we as a society become so dependent on drugs? Is it the ease of obtaining them? Is it the belief of "a pill for every ill"? Do we want a quick fix? Have we been programmed by all the commercials we cannot avoid whenever we turn on our TV? The upside of all these drug commercials is we have been made aware of the many side effects all these drugs have. It is my experience that side effects are barely discussed during the doctor appointment. Could this be because most appointments only last an average of 20 minutes, leaving no time for an in depth discussion? Even when we do not see an improvement in our health condition, we find ourselves going back to the doctor. Is there any other industry we "trust" so much? Have we been brainwashed to "trust" our doctor?

Have you ever heard of Integrative Medicine or Functional Medicine? Interestingly enough I became familiar with Integrative Medicine when I was introduced to network marketing by a Defeat Autism Now doctor. The first Integrative doctor I met was led to practice this way because of his own health challenges. I find this scenario very often with the out of box practitioners my work has led me too. All of them had a health challenge that allopathic medicine could not treat which led them to discover a treatment on their own.

Many years went by before I too developed skepticism when it came to allopathic medicine. Here are the following experiences that led to my confidence being eroded: It started with my Autism Spectrum journey with my oldest daughter when I was told by my daughter's pediatrician that she will grow out of her ear infections. She did not grow out of her ear infections. In fact she had two sets of tubes over many years. The significant scarring that resulted from this procedure led to a tympanoplasty in one ear upon entering high school. I have since learned that a chiropractor would have been a much better way to treat ear infections. I also had a pediatrician tell me in close proximity to my youngest daughter receiving vaccines and beginning to exhibit asthmatic symptoms that she was just experiencing "temporary asthma" I now know that this was from the vaccines and this was a contraindication to receiving anymore. Incidentally this pediatrician now prides himself in specializing in asthma and is not vaccine friendly. My middle daughter suffered from severe gastrointestinal distress at times after vaccine administration. After a complete work up at a Children's Hospital I was told by this pediatrician that since they were not able to find a cause, her severe pain was all in my daughter's mind. I now know that the pain that she suffered was real and was caused by dysbiosis. This is the upset of the natural balance of micro-organisms in your gut.

I myself had some experiences with family practitioners that raised some red flags in my mind. I was told that swollen ankles was a sign of getting old (I was only in my forties). I know this is not true because after I discovered Living Alkalized Water, which I will talk about in a future chapter, this problem has been resolved. I also went to another family practitioner because of symptoms of menopause.

This doctor was ready to prescribe a synthetic hormone knowing a side effect is cancer. When I asked her about this she said "yes that is a side effect." When I told her I would not be taking that drug she wrote in my chart that I was going against medical advice. WOW!

Hospital

Another way to stay in our greatness is to avoid the hospital as a patient at all costs. If a hospital stay is needed always have a family member or friend present. Patient harm from hospitals may be the 3rd leading cause of death. According to the Journal of Patient Safety, which is a peer reviewed medical journal, 440 000 deaths a year are linked to medical error. If you have to go to the hospital never go alone. As of June 2015 the American College of Emergency Physicians policy includes referring out under vaccinated emergency department patients. This policy allows for patients who cannot be referred out for any reason to be vaccinated in the emergency room. The policy states that appropriate education (ie. Center For Disease Control Vaccination Statement) must be given to the patient prior to administration of the vaccine. I find this a bit comical if this was not so serious because the CDC is currently under investigation by the United States Congress for alleged fraud. In light of this I would think anything that was given out by the CDC should be under scrutiny. I would also highly recommend the patient ask for the vaccine insert prior to any vaccine administration so they get the true picture when it comes to all the ingredients and contraindications.

The last time I was in the hospital was a very negative experience for me. I was sent there by my doctor as an outpatient to get a CT scan to rule out a tumor in my lungs. At this time I had been suffering from bronchitis for over two months. After the CT scan was performed I was told I was going to be admitted. To this day I do not know why I did not fight harder against this. It could be because I was under a lot of stress having just lost a very close friend in a car accident days before. When I voiced my opposition to the doctor he implied that if I left I would be leaving against medical advice. I started thinking about insurance and the possibility of lack of coverage should I leave against medical advice. Next thing I know I am being told I am going to be getting an echocardiogram. I did not understand what this procedure had to do with my current health condition. At that point I was under their spell and too emotionally exhausted to fight. Since my intention was never to be admitted I also had come alone. Thankfully the following morning I told them I was fine and left with another prescription for a proton pump inhibitor to treat my GERD (Gastroesophageal Reflux Disease).

My second negative hospital experience involved visiting my mother-in- law in the hospital. She had been admitted for atrial fibrillation as a result of a reaction from a drug called genique gel that she had just been given to treat incontinence. While I was in the room this young doctor came into the room and told my mother-in-law that he wanted to perform an ablation procedure on her heart. I heard her tell the doctor that she did not want an ablation procedure. I was very happy that she had decided against this. I have the belief that any procedure where money is at play should be fully researched before giving it consideration. Fast forward to the following morning and my mother-in-law was calling my husband to let him know they were prepping her for the ablation procedure. This was the first time that the family had heard anything of this. The stunning thing to me was learning that a doctor can return to the patient's room after the family member has left and bully the patient into agreeing to a procedure that she knew nothing about. Unfortunately for me I was only an in-law so my hands were tied. Within 3 weeks my mother-in-law had passed away from a hospital acquired infection called pneumonia. I found out this is quite common. According to the CDC as of April 2014 hospital acquired infections now affect 1 in 25 patients. The most common infections are in the blood stream, urinary tract, surgical site, and pneumonia (including pneumonia acquired from a ventilator).

In my mind all I have to do is look at the food and drinks that are served to the patients in the hospital and that is my first clue that this setting is not about the wellness that we are striving for and our body is crying for as a patient. The electromagnetic field that you are surrounded by there is also very suspect.

When you go to a hospital today you will also notice nurses that wear a mask and nurses that do not. The ones that wear a mask are not willing to be vaccinated. There is even a movement in hospitals to vaccinate nurses and fire them from their job if they do not comply. Nurses who are pregnant are being told a vaccine is safe even when the vaccine insert itself states the safety and efficacy for women who are pregnant has NOT been established. It goes even further and says we also do not know if this vaccine can impact fertility. According to the VAERS (Vaccine Adverse Events Report) website there have been 4,168 fetal deaths from the flu shot in the first trimester. This could very well be a contributing factor to the "nursing shortage" that appears to be ongoing. This medical freedom battle that is going on between the hospital administration and their staff can only be an impediment to the care the patients receive in the hospital.

Cancer

I could not write a chapter on Sickcare and Healthcare without covering the topic of that dreaded C word: CANCER. I think we have been programmed to fear cancer. When we hear those words "You have only (fill in the blank here) months to live" our brain goes into a state of panic and fear which can lead to historic mistakes. Yes cancer is a disease that is caused by dehydration, inflammation, oxidative stress, and acidosis. There is definitely an emotional component in play as well, which the "doctors" take full advantage of and totally ignore at the same time in regard to how it relates to the state of sickness in the body. Negative emotions can cause very acidic conditions in the body. You can see this in a blood cell analysis. Blood cell analysis can reveal a lot to you about what is going on in regard to health condition of your cells which are the building blocks of your body. There are two places in my surrounding area currently where I can take advantage of this amazing technology! You can sometimes find this technology in a wellness center such as a health food store. It is interesting to note that if you go back in history microscopes were common place at one time in rooms where patients were seen. I look at the blood like gas in your car. When you see blood cells in an acidic condition, the cells are all clumped together and have lost their shape and buoyancy. When you see this live in action you get an understanding of maybe why you are feeling sick and why your organs are not functioning to their full potential. Everything in our body is connected and I believe many "specialists" out there are not applying this to how they are practicing medicine.

As I was researching this topic I thought it would be interesting to look into when oncology actually became a specialty. Oncology became a subspecialty of internal medicine in 1972. Last year alone 1600 people a day died of cancer in the United States. In one year 120 billion dollars is made alone on cancer!!! The income of an oncologist is the fastest growing income in the medical field. Having been myself in the field of network marketing since 2009 I see a lot of resemblance in how the oncology field operates. What I mean by that is the oncologist himself purchases and profits from any of the various drugs he chooses to buy at wholesale. The only difference is instead of marking up his product to his customer as in network marketing he marks up his drugs and passes it on to his patients insurance company. His livelihood depends on whether he sells you his drugs. Because he is a " doctor" he is given even more power by being allowed to medically claim "If you do not do this you are going to die". Now let us review again what kind of state your brain is in when you initially go and visit your oncologist whom you have never met. I will repeat again, historic mistakes are made when we go into fear and panic. Do oncologists have the right setting to capitalize on your fear for their livelihood? The answer to that question is an emphatic YES!!! Of course they do. How many professionals in their field can say "if you do not do what I say you are going to die?" What is most alarming is if you have cancer your allopathic doctor is not allowed to prescribe any treatment other than surgery, chemo, or radiation or their own profession who espouses "do no harm" will have their license revoked.

It is their way or the highway in this model. Thankfully we now have some doctors/healers taking the highway. What makes this even more remarkable is that American doctors cannot offer any other advice in regard to lifestyle choices unless it is recommended in tandem with their conventional FDA approved treatment. My advice to anyone that finds themselves having to seek consul over a cancer diagnosis is to come to their appointment armed with independent research. Yes you are not a "doctor" who has learned about drugs and procedures that go hand in hand with their healing model. However, it is important to remember this is your body and brain and it works very well if it is able to recognize and process what goes into it and it is not frozen in fear. What is even most important to realize is that our mindset is even more powerful than our body when it comes to healing and is in our full control and can be adjusted at will at any time. I believe the emotional toll inside the body that is accompanied with this disease condition is a major contributing factor to causing more cancer and lowering the cellular voltage even further. It is a time to bring structure into chaos. It is a time to visualize the beautiful healthy body we were destined to have. It is a time to practice self-talk and empower ourselves to calm our brain from the fear and panic of the unknown. The worst thing about cancer is not the "cancer". It is about how your cancer is being treated for financial gain. If you hear those words " you have only (fill in the blank) months to live" realize that in this moment in time you will now begin to live!!! Find and embrace the healing power you have within. It is there!

ADHD and Psychology/Psychiatry

In my journey to seek wellness for my youngest daughter I found myself in the office of a psychiatrist to whom we were referred by a psychologist. I learned there is a cozy relationship between a psychologist and a psychiatrist. One diagnoses and the other prescribes the drugs.

If you recall in my introductory chapter my youngest daughter received her ADHD diagnosis after a 15 minute conversation with her pediatrician. It was her school counselor and her positive ADHD results on the Connor Rating Scale that led us to this office visit. At no time was there any attempt to rule out anything physical going on inside her body and/or brain like ordering a blood test or a brain scan. The first psychiatrist lasted a few months with the last visit being passed off to his assistant. The last visit included being handed a sample of Respiradal which, as I write this, has law suits being filed all over the country. By this time we have been on the drug merry go round for awhile and I was getting very weary. I knew before I decided to give my daughter this drug I needed to go home and research it. I became alarmed at what I was learning in regard to the side effects of this drug and decided I needed to find a new psychiatrist. We tried a few more meds, one at a time, with the new psychiatrist but the meltdowns continued and I became more disillusioned. The following is a list of the sleep meds and psychotropic drugs my daughter was on at various times from 2nd grade until middle school: Strattera, Focalin, Ritalin, Adderal (which is now being characterized as crystal meth) Ritalin, Trazodone, Clonidine, and Mirtazapine. Despite them all, no improvement was noted in her sleep and behavior. I did have the unfortunate experience of seeing her put on a sleep medication in tandem with a psychotropic medication and she immediately became bipolar. It was really scary to see and I knew to stop the medication right away after consulting with the Nurse Practitioner in the Developmental Pediatricians office. I was shocked that the Nurse Practitioner had no knowledge of what could happen when these two kinds of drugs are taken together. I was really upset. This specialist also gives these medications to children. Knowing what I know now about drugs which are acidic, toxic, and dehydrating why would I even think this would improve "ADHD" long term? ADHD is already an indicator of a toxic condition in the body and brain. The last thing I want to do is increase the toxicity load not to mention what these drugs can do to harm the heart.

I thought it would be interesting to look at the history of ADHD as a diagnosis. In order for a psychiatrist to come up with the diagnosis for his patient he refers to the Diagnostic and Statistical Manual of Mental Disorders (DSM) which was written for the first time in 1952. Sixteen years later in 1968 the second DSM came out and it was here that ADHD was recognized for the first time under the name of Hyper Kinetic Impulse Disorder. Twelve more years would go by when the DSM-3 would come out. In 1980 Hyper Kinetic Impulse Disorder would become Attention Deficit Disorder, only this time it would also include two subtypes: ADD with Hyperactivity and ADD without Hyperactivity. It is also interesting to note that in 1986 our Government passed the National Childhood Vaccine Injury Act which was a no fault compensation program. The was done because the drug manufacturers were becoming liable for the harm that the DTP vaccine was causing and as a result parents were filing many lawsuits and drug companies were beginning to pull out of the vaccine business. It was at this time that the drug companies transferred their liability to the Federal Government. At the same time this Act was passed the Center for Disease Control put together a Vaccine Information Statement for every vaccine that were now being given to parents prior to their child being vaccinated. These statements, which are still used today, are in no way indicative of what can actually occur to a susceptible immunocompromised population. One size DOES NOT fit all. If you are considering this procedure a look at the vaccine insert is what I highly recommend.

In 1987 the DSM-3 was revised and the subtypes of ADHD were eliminated and it just became called ADHD. In the year 2000 they came out with the 4th edition which went back to subtypes and added an additional one: Combined type ADHD, Predominately Inattentive type ADHD, and Predominately Hyperactive-Impulsive type ADHD. Oddly enough within 4 years of the National Childhood Vaccine Injury Act coming into play, which absolved the drug manufacturers of all liability, many more vaccines appeared on the schedule and we also saw a very significant increase in allergies, asthma, ADHD, and Autism. This is NOT A COINCIDENCE!!! It saddens me to see what the psychiatrists have done to our population, in particular the children.

There are currently at least 11 commonly used psychotropic medications used for ADHD. According to the IMS Health, a company that provides information services and technology for the healthcare industry, 8,389,034 kids ranging from 0 to 17 years were on psychiatric drugs in the year 2013. Every week a child goes into a coma from a psychotropic drug. Every month 4 children die from psychiatric drug side effects. Every week a child commits suicide. Twelve regulatory drug agencies have issued warnings on stimulants (ie. Ritalin) for causing addiction, insomnia, mania, depression, psychosis, heart problems, sudden death, and stroke. One Hundred seventy two drug regulatory warnings and studies show antidepressant use leads to hallucination, aggression, hostility, violence, homicidal thoughts, and suicide. Drug regulatory agencies from seven countries including the US warn that anti-psychotic drugs can cause death yet they are prescribed to toddlers. It is my hope that there will be a movement sooner rather than later away from the drugs and toward a holistic healing approach.

Dentistry

I wanted to cover the dental profession because this is also interfering with our greatness. Their procedures include an applied neurotoxin as well as a sample they give you to take home. What am I talking about? I am talking about a fluoride treatment and toothpaste. Fluoride is a standard procedure that they put on your teeth at the end of a teeth cleaning. The toothpaste they give you to take home more than likely contains fluoride.

Let us go back to the year 2006. In November 2006 the American Dental Association sent out an email to its members recommending that parents use no or low fluoride water to make infant formula. The Center for the Disease Control soon issued the same warning but neither of these sources informed the public at large. In 2011 a panel under the American Dental Association Council of Scientific Affairs backtracked stating parents may use water with fluoride but should be on the lookout for the possibility of enamel fluorosis. This causes defects in the tooth enamel. If this is a concern fluoride free water is recommended. In 2012 a Harvard study came out showing fluoride water reduces children's IQ. This is just one of many studies out there. Why has this not yet been accepted by the scientific community? This denial is reflective of the same inaction we see in regard to taking mercury out of the vaccines. The same journal the Lancet that removed Dr. Wakefield's paper linking gastrointestinal disease to the MMR vaccine officially classified fluoride as a developmental neurotoxin in 2014. Did you know that the World Health Organization puts fluoride in the same category as arsenic on the naturally occurring hazard list? What is a neurotoxin? A neurotoxin is poison that can harm tissues in the brain, spinal cord, and nervous system. The most detrimental time that it can harm the brain in child development is pre-birth and early childhood. Fluoride lowers IQ. Fluoride and aluminum may have an active role in the Alzheimer's connection. When aluminum comes in contact with fluoride it attaches itself and becomes aluminum fluoride and bypasses the blood brain barrier. The one thing we do know is fluoride and aluminum have a synergistic effect which means only a small amount of either metal is needed for toxicity to occur.

Here are some other alarming facts about fluoride. It doubles the risk of hypothyroidism. Degeneration of the brain can occur. I saw this with my own eyes in my late father's diagnosis which coincidentally had the word degeneration in it. I will go into this in more detail in a later chapter. Fluoride also compromises the pineal gland where melatonin is made. Think of the pineal gland as the light switch for melatonin. If you turn on the light in the middle of the night your melatonin production shuts off and does not come back on. When you disrupt your sleep at night your body stops repairing itself. Fluoride also increases the danger of lead poisoning. Fluoride may also be linked to ADHD. Did you know fluoride is in antidepressant medication? WOW! The medications that contain fluoride are Prozac, Paxil, Zoloft, and Lexapro. I find this very ironic because fluoride can cause depression which is what these medications are supposed to treat!

I cannot talk about dentistry without mentioning mercury amalgams. This is a procedure that is going on all over the country. It is on my list to get done because mercury actually emits a vapor every time you chew. I have heard someone say they stopped aging once they had their mercury fillings removed. There is a lot of preparation that both the patient, dentist and his staff have to do before this procedure can even be implemented. Here is how a friend described it: "What was most notable was the preparation for the removal - what the staff had to wear and what I had to wear before the procedure could even begin. I liken it to hazmat suits. Head coverings, body coverings, special glasses and full face, filtered masks for the staff. Head covering, clothing covering, isolating the teeth and a dam to block off the rest of my mouth while the teeth were being worked on. Then there was the special vacuum unit to suck out the vapors."

Chances are if you have a chronic disease there is most likely a dental infection lurking. Believe it or not dentists may even have more of an influence on your health than your doctor! I find it fascinating to know that every one of our teeth is wired into an acupuncture meridian. Whatever happens to the tooth happens to the meridian.

The meridian is a wire with multiple organs including a tooth on the same circuit. So if you have a tooth infection the corresponding organs of that tooth is also affected. This most likely was not taught in Medical School or Dental School.

CHAPTER 5
AUTISM AKA VACCINE INDUCED BRAIN INJURY

Current Vaccine Schedule

This latest list of recommendations of vaccines for the year 2016 by the CDC from birth thru 18 years makes me want to cry. Are moms and dads in our country really handing their beautiful babies over to the pediatrician's office and allowing 7 vaccines at a time to be injected in their babies blood at the 6th month "Well Child Visit"? This was the same amount of injections required in 1983 from birth thru 18 years of age!!! In the year 2016 the CDC is recommending 50 injections from birth thru 18 years of age!!! Has our immune system, that are creator made, become so inadequate over 33 years that we have to triple the amount of vaccines at each "Well Child Visit" since 1983? My oldest daughter was born in 1989 and I can guarantee you I did not leave the pediatricians office with any more than 2 band aids or plasters as they say in England. I recently saw a photo on Facebook of very young twins and they each had 3 band aids on each of their leg. What? Let's talk about what we are seeing in many children who get vaccinated.

We are seeing very high fevers, rashes and/or big red welts all over the body, hard knots at the injection site, eczema, droopy half faces, crooked smiles, no more talking, blank stares, no eye contact, chronic diarrhea, nonstop high pitched screaming for days, arched backs, seizures, severe constipation, chronic ear infections, allergies, asthma, cancer and death..... the list goes on. A word on the nonstop high pitched scream; Dr. Russell Blaylock, a former Neurosurgeon and now a researcher, has named this the encephalitic scream. What is happening here is the child's brain is swelling and is pressing against the skull. When this happens the parents will contact the doctor and be told this is normal and the baby will be better tomorrow. This is a TOTAL LIE!!! There is nothing normal about brain inflammation!!!

Live Viruses

Did you know that vaccines with live viruses or bacteria carry a risk for patients actually getting the disease itself? Also did you know that the weakened vaccine strain live virus can mutate and get stronger which can cause serious complications from vaccine strain viral infections? Which vaccines that are on the schedule now are made from live viruses? These vaccines are the chicken pox (Varicella), Measles (MMR), Rotavirus, Flu-nasal spray, and shingles. So the first live virus your child gets is in the Rotavirus vaccine at two and four months. According to the CDC if you are getting the Rotateq version of this vaccine you get another one at 6 months. There are two versions. How they decide who gets what version would be a good question to ask. Also the flu vaccine is also on the 6 month schedule which could include another live virus should you get the nasal spray form. At 12 months your child gets two vaccines which contain a live virus, the chicken pox and the measles. Fast forward to the 50 and up population when you are now eligible to receive the shingles vaccine. If you get the flu mist at the same time you now have given your body two live viruses. There are several contraindications for the flu mist vaccine according to the CDC.

1. Allergy to any components of the vaccine itself
2. Children age 2-17 years of age receiving aspirin or aspirin containing products
3. Egg allergy
4. Pregnant women
5. Immunosuppressed
6. Age 2-4years old with asthma or wheezing in the past 12 months
7. Taken antiviral medication in previous 48 hours

There are another 28 pages of contraindications should you like to see more. I myself have seen enough.

After learning this I do have very good news however. I have learned on the Mayo Clinic website the name of the blood test that can tell you if your child is immunosuppressed. The name of this test is Immunoglobulins IgA, IgG, and IgM. This was the test I heard a chiropractor who specialized in the brain talk about at the Family Cafe which is a yearly state conference held for families with children of disabilities. The IgA looks at the mucous membrane. The IgG looks at all body fluids. The IgM looks at the body and lymph fluid. Since the live virus of these vaccines are being injected into the blood of our children this sounds like a very necessary test that we need to ask our pediatrician to do PRIOR to vaccination.

Now let us take a look at all the testing they do to make sure all these vaccines that they are injecting in the blood at the same time are not causing HARM. The only testing that is being done on the vaccines are being done by parties who financially benefit from vaccine sales. No long term tests have been done! The experiment that many of us are willingly taking part in because we 'trust our doctor" is taking place TODAY.

Amygdala and Aspergers

I did find one vaccine study involving monkeys. The study was published in 2010. Twelve boy, baby monkeys were given vaccines according to the US vaccination schedule. The study showed that the MMR ,DTaP, and HIB vaccinated primates had significantly altered amygdala growth compared to the 4 unvaccinated primates. The vaccinated monkeys also showed a significant increase in total brain volume. This is consistent with the total brain volume that we see in children with "Autism" between 6 and 14 months of age.[5] I am reminded this may be why we see head circumferences being measured during the "Well Child Visit". What is the amygdala and what does it do? The amygdala gives you the ability to feel certain emotions and recognize them in other people. It is located in the limbic system of your brain. The less active your limbic system is the more positive a person you are. It is also related to bonding. Stress activates your limbic system. This is also where smell is processed which means there is a direct correlation with what you smell and how you feel. The amygdala is the emotion you feel before you take action. It controls your fear and anxiety.

[5] Miller, Neil Z. Miller's Review of Critical Vaccine Studies: 400 Important Scientific Papers Summarized for Parents and Researchers. Sante Fe: New Atlantean, 2016. Print.

When I see what is happening with the young people out there this makes total sense to me. This sure fits the former Aspergers's diagnosis that is no longer recognized as of May 2013 in the DSM-5 but now falls under the umbrella term of Autism Spectrum Disorder. I believe this is an attempt to normalize this population which I find really tragic. Some of the characteristics of Asperger's is difficulty with social skills and anxiety which go hand in hand. Struggling with social skills can definitely correlate with anxiety. Humans are not meant to be alone. If you fail socially time and time again it becomes very difficult to go on without a lot of support. According to a blog on the American Association of Christian Counselors website which has 50,000 members, "the rates of suicide are rising among teens with high functioning Autism (formerly called Asperger's/Aspies). There is not a study to provide empirical numbers, but those working with Aspie teens say they are at a 40-50% higher risk of completing suicide than their Neuro-typical (NT) counterparts." Another unpublished analysis of medical records of more than 2,000 California adults with "Autism" found that 1.8 percent of these individuals attempted suicide between 2008 and 2012, compared with 0.3 percent of controls.[6] The way things stand now it looks like these numbers will only go up unless we as a society wake up and take control of our own health. Everyone deserves to have successful social and romantic relationships, become independent, and obtain meaningful work with a purpose. I believe embracing personal development and entrepreneurship will be a shining light for this population which I am excited to write about in a later chapter.

---

[6] "Spectrum | Autism Research New and Opinion." Spectrum. Web. 02 Mar.2016

Herd Immunity

I would like to talk about herd immunity and the greater good. We hear this all the time in defense of vaccines. In fact the state of CA has decided as of July 2016 personal and religious exemptions in public schools, private schools, and daycares will no longer be accepted which includes kids who already have a vaccine induced brain injury. The parent's only option is to home school; this is how much importance they put on "herd immunity".

First of all vaccination is not the same as immunization. The definition of the word immune is having a high degree of resistance to a disease. So if you have a high degree of resistance to a disease that means you will not get the disease. The definition of immunization according to Wikipedia is the process by which an individual's immune system becomes fortified against an agent. Vaccination is not the same as immunization at all because it does not make you become resistant to a disease. If it did all these vaccine boosters would not be necessary. Also there would not be a fear of unvaccinated people. The baby boomers who received a miniscule amount of vaccines compared to today's schedule have long since lost their immunity and there has not been a rise in communicable diseases in their population.

The original theory of herd immunity was based on a belief from an observation and came during a time when there were no vaccinations. In 1933 a physician in Baltimore noticed that if 68% of children younger than 15 years old already had the measles and recovered, the rest of the population was protected from getting it

NATURALLY. The physician's study was published in the May 1933 American Journal of Epidemiology. In 1967 the United States Public Health Service used this same idea, applied it to vaccinations by increasing the percentage needed to be vaccinated for measles even further, but the herd immunity that they expected did not occur. Today they have raised the herd immunity percentage even higher to 95% and yet herd immunity evades them because vaccine induced immunity is not natural immunity. We are bypassing our immune system by not allowing these diseases.

For proof that live virus vaccines shed you only have to go to the St. Jude Children's Hospital website and read the following warnings:

Do not allow people to visit your child if:

- They have received oral polio or smallpox vaccines within 4 weeks.
- They have received the nasal flu vaccine within 1 week; or
- They have rashes after receiving the chickenpox (Varicella) vaccine or MMR (Measles, Mumps, Rubella) vaccine.

When I read this I ask myself how many school children are passing these live viruses on to their classmates and yet many want to attack the unvaccinated. How many of these children are immunosuppressed and have no knowledge of it? Who is being harmed then?

Nagalase

What I am about to tell you is very controversial but I believe with all my being to be very true. I would be very neglectful not to mention this. Have you heard of all the very mysterious deaths of doctors coming out of Florida in the last several months beginning in June of last year with the sudden death of Dr. Bradstreet, and followed by many alternative medicine doctors in other states? Most likely you are not aware of this because our news is very selected these days because Big Pharma has control of the media. Many of these doctor/healers had three things in common.

1. They all learned about a substance called Nagalase that is being injected into the body through immunization.
2. They all had their offices raided by the FDA and accused of using GCMAF.
3. They all had a close working relationship with Dr. Bradstreet. At the time Dr. Bradstreet, who was world renown, was working extensively with treating Autism and finding out the why.

It is my understanding that this information has been out for awhile. What is Nagalase and what is it doing to the body? Nagalase is an enzyme protein that is made by cancer cells and viruses. When Nagalase is introduced to the body it causes immunodeficiency. It was the opinion of all these doctors that Nagalase is being introduced to the body through immunization. This discovery began when Dr. Bradstreet found super high concentrations of Nagalase in his children with Autism. The reason Nagalase causes immunodeficiency is because it blocks the human GCMAF (Globulin component

Macrophage Activating Factor) production. Let us break this down. The GC protein in our body combined with macrophages, which are the systems vacuum cleaners, kill the cancer cells and stop the cytokine storms. The cytokine storms come from chemicals that are produced by the macrophages. Cytokines cause inflammation and the more cytokines the more insulin resistance. Also when the macrophages do not get enough Vitamin D they let go of large amounts of cytokines. This is where Nagalase comes into play. Nagalase debilitates the GC protein so it can no longer attach to Vitamin D. The body cannot make GCMAF without Vitamin D. GCMAF is the body's single most effective way to kill virus and cancer cells. This is how Nagalase destroys the immune system.

Since the human GCMAF was compromised by the Nagalase in Dr. Bradstreet's patients with Autism he obtained GCMAF from a lab in Europe. When he was able to give 1100 patients GCMAF his response rate was 85%!!! On the bell curve 15% of the patients showed total eradication of symptoms!!! This lab in Europe has since disappeared.[7]

There are currently 59 research papers on GCMAF. 20 of these papers are related to cancer. 46 of these papers can be accessed online. GCMAF is the lifeline of our immune system. When Nagalase goes into the blood by way of a vaccine injection the body's ability to make GCMAF and kill cancer cells is shut down.

---

[7] Noakes, David. "Age of Autism." Age of Autism. Web. 02 Mar. 2016. "GCMAF For the Treatment of Cancer, Autism, Inflammation, Viral, and Bacterial Disease"

Dr. Bradstreet found that out of 800 cases of children with Autism, 80% were found to have Nagalase. He suspected undiagnosed, undetected cancer in this population.[8]

The latest research in diabetes shows that macrophage activity can have an added drawback. Macrophages at work produce chemicals called cytokines. Cytokines cause inflammation and compromises insulin action in the liver and muscle. Diabetes 2 displays higher cytokines which leads to more insulin resistance. A cytokine storm can also occur when macrophages do not get significant quantities of Vitamin D. The Nagalase is causing the failure of Vitamin D to do its job which is to attach to the macrophage. When you have less Vitamin D the macrophages are in a more active state. When Vitamin D cannot attach itself to the macrophage a cytokine storm ensues in phosphotase which also increases inflammation in the cardiovascular system leading to heart disease, athroscelerotic plaqueing and diabetes. The end result is dying earlier than you normally would.[9]

The Gut

So now you know how the immune system is being compromised, let us talk about the gut which is the immune system and our second brain. In the major gut diseases we also see a deficiency in Vitamin D.

---

[8]HackenLively, Ken. "Age of Autism" Age of Autism. Web. 02 Mar.2016. "Dr. Bradstreet, Nagalease, Viral Issue in Autism"

[9]Hawkins, Meredith, and Prettie Kishor. "Diabetes ForecastA The Healthy Living Magazine." Diabetes Forecast. Web.02 Mar. 2016. "The Role of Vitamin D and Type 2 Diabetes"

Our gut is also the microbiome, where are good and bad bacteria live. Did you know we also have neurotransmitters in our gut? So many times our gut talks to us but are we listening? I should have listened to my gut when I took my youngest in to the pediatrician, having just arrived from living abroad. It did not feel right to me when the nurse at the pediatrician's office told me I now have to sign off on the vaccines before they are given. The reason people have you sign something is more likely than not for liability reasons which should have given me pause. What are they hiding that I do not know about? Now I know....... we are talking about the gut brain connection. I am thankful allopathic medicine is starting to study what we Autism moms have figured out long ago. When a smart lady who I met at my daughter's school, that did the academic testing suggested I take my daughter off of sugar, dyes, preservatives, additives, and basically eat from our foods natural source I could see improvement. Sugar really caused her brain to act like she was on heroin. It was unreal and very scary to watch. There is a direct correlation between blood sugar and brain inflammation. The way to combat brain inflammation is to stay away from carbohydrates and eat good fats. The opposite of what the United States Department of Agriculture (USDA) food pyramid has told us all these years. We really are what we eat!

Cellular Voltage

The one book that I have read that stands alone from all the others is Dr. Jerry Tennant's book "Healing Is Voltage," it is in its 3rd edition!!! This was my first introduction to cellular voltage and I cannot get enough of it. This is a key piece to how our body really works. Our body is a vibrating machine. Not only does the body vibrate but everything around the body vibrates too! Allopathic medicine has a lot of catching up to do. There is no doubt in our grandparent's day it was easier to keep our voltage up. The electromagnetic field was minimal compared to today. In order for our cells to repair the voltage it needs to be at -50mV. There are many ways to raise our voltage. The five ways I will mention now are light, living water, color, sound, and essential oils.

Let us talk about light first. Interestingly enough in the late 19th to mid -20th Century, sunlight therapy or heliotherapy as it was called was considered to be the gold standard treatment for infectious diseases in Europe. This was the treatment before the age of antibiotic drugs. The studies showed the many healing features of the sun in dramatically lowering blood pressure, decreasing cholesterol, lowering blood sugar and increasing the number of white blood cells.

Dr. Auguste Rollier, a medical doctor and author, was known as the most famous heliotherapist of all. At the height of his career he operated 36 clinics with over 1,000 beds in Leysin, Switzerland. He chose locations that were 5,000 feet above sea level so his patients would have access to as much UV light as possible. It is funny how this is the light we were warned about, beginning in the 1980's, to stay away from when the toxic sunscreen campaign began. Even sunglasses block out the critical rays of the light spectrum which the body needs to function. The full spectrum light of the sun does not only go to your eyes, it also goes to the hypothalamus in your brain. The hypothalamus is the command center for your circadian rhythm (body clock).

It may be surprising to know that our body is 75% water!!! Drinking living, alkaline, antioxidant water from an ionizer is another way to raise our voltage in our body. Our water needs to have the property of being an electron donor. Acid water, reverse osmosis, distilled water, and bottled water are all electron stealers. In my journey to wellness I came upon this living alkaline ionized water. The filtration system in this ionizer removes everything but fluoride. A pre-filter system to remove fluoride is advised should this be present in your water. This new ionizer technology also has the ability to recalibrate the source water according to the pH. Another exciting feature is the chip technology which allows for upgrades as they become available. Gone are the days when you have to buy a brand new machine to upgrade.

When this water comes out of the hose it looks cloudy, which is an indicator that hydrogen is present. My favorite part is watching the initial bubble movement after it is poured in the glass. This is exactly why it is so powerful! When living water goes into the body its properties flush everything out! There are some natural settings left where this pure water can be found around the world. This water gets its charge as it flows over the mineral rich rocks.

Since water has frequency I wonder if this is why we find so many missing kids with Autism drowned in bodies of water close to their home. The definition of frequency is the rate in which a vibration occurs that constitutes a wave. Are these kids with Autism seeking a higher frequency for their body? I believe this is related.

Frequency can be raised with color too! Each color is a different frequency and relates differently to your individual cells. The color you see and the color you are wearing is vibrating. I have a personal example I would like to share. I bought these lime green patterned holey jeans because they were my company color at the time. EVERYTIME I wear them I get many compliments throughout the day and everyone wants to know where to get them! I know this is because of the color combined with my own vibrations because interestingly enough that color signifies healing and that coincides with my passion to lead everyone that has been harmed by the medical establishment to healing! There is even a science about this called chromotherapy which uses colors to adjust body vibrations to frequencies that result in health and harmony!

Sound is one of my favorite ways to raise my frequency. Listening to words with music can even be more healing. Sound can either lower or raise our frequency. For example I have a difficult time listening to a bass sound that has a steady beat especially in the morning. I find it jarring to my body. I also recall being at my niece's wedding and toward the end I could not take the sound of the band anymore. I found it exhausting! Some of the baby boomers remember what the sound of fingernails on a chalk board was like. This is a frequency that sends chills down most spines. I also know there are people whose body experience pain when they hear the sound of a fire drill. I have also listened to music that has immediately brought me to tears, I surprised myself. It is very powerful when that happens. We have all experienced a time when hearing a beautiful voice has given us chills. All these examples are our cells vibrating to the sounds that we hear and the emotions that we feel. We also at any one time have emotions with frequency that we are hiding in our cells. Words and our emotions can raise and lower our frequency too!

I think it may be time with all the noise we are bombarded with daily to take an inventory of the sounds that surround us and separate from the ones that lower our frequency. I use to always think I needed the radio on to keep my brain alert. When I made the decision to stop listening to it I found I could hear my thoughts much more clearly in the quiet. I believe God, in my case, or a higher power speaks to us in the quiet.

What do you do when you hear negativity? Do you keep listening to it and bring yourself down or do you excuse yourself? I know a very successful guy who will leave if the environment he is in is bringing him down. You may need to ask whomever to please be more positive. There may be times during your day where you want more control in your environment and you put your phone on silent or chose to wear earphones. Be aware of what you say to others with your words, tone, and volume. Are you raising or lowering their cell frequency? Make your goal to raise the frequency of the room higher than when you came in.

Have you ever heard of the word earthing? I first became aware of earthing in a former network marketing company I was in. They felt it was important enough to post a book called "Earthing" on their website which, upon further investigation, I purchased. It was interesting to note this book was co-authored by Dr. Stephen Sinatra who is a cardiologist and a FORMER speaker for Big Pharma. Dr. Sinatra is my go to doctor for the heart! His website is heartmdinstitute.com

I think my first experience with earthing unbeknownst to me was walking around barefoot in the grass as a child living in Illinois. I do not believe we sprayed our grass with pesticides back then. Now living in Florida, the only opportunity to really earth is to walk on the sidewalk, garden with bare hands, or my favorite walking on the beach. There is a reason we experience calmness when we ground our body to the earth. When we cannot ground we are separated from the healing energy of the earth.

Our Amazing Brain

I believe as children have become more developmentally delayed so have we seen an increase in bullying. I can definitely understand why. When a child sees a classmate not looking at him while he is talking to him he feels ignored. When a child is slow to follow a conversation his classmates are having they may react by teasing him. Many times teachers find themselves having to repeat things over and over and the struggling child becomes frustrated and feels dumb. This has everything to do with the pathways of the brain. The website brainhighways.com gave me a great understanding of this. These are brilliant videos because the kids are the teachers. It is interesting that "Autism" is not even mentioned on this website because this mimics exactly what is going on with this population.

I would like to go back to the topic lack of eye contact. I came upon an article on Yahoo.com today where they ask kids why they cannot or do not maintain eye contact. Here are the highlights of what these kids said that I found most intriguing and confirmed to me again that movement is key to recovering "Autism".

"It's a constant stream of extra sensory or processing information on top of what I'm already trying to sort through in my head. It can disrupt any thought or speaking process I have going on and zaps my energy quickly." -Laura

"My eyes take pictures of the things I see, and I can mentally go back and revisit these pictures in my mind for a very long time, I become overcome with so many pictures of your eyes, it is overwhelming, and I have to look away to give my mind something else to process." -Sydney

"It can feel like you're standing there naked. It's very difficult to form a coherent thought with all of this going on in your head. My trick for making eye contact more bearable is to make 'eye contact' with peoples' eyebrows. Nobody ever knows the difference." -Megan

"For me, it's difficult because I feel like the person I'm making eye contact with may be able to see just how socially awkward and odd I am. I force myself to make eye contact when speaking to a person, but it can actually make my eyes burn or water while doing it." -Jill

"When I make eye contact, the world around me blocks out. I can only process the immense pain and discomfort that comes to my brain. This pain goes if I look away" -Lucy

"If I try to look at you when I'm trying to say something I have a hard time getting what I want to say out because I can't separate the processing that takes place with both tasks." -Rosie

"As a child, I didn't give any eye contact at all, but I now give it in certain situations and not others. If I'm stressed about something, I likely won't be giving any eye contact. A lot of the time it feels spooky. It feels as though someone is looking right into your very soul. That's why it used to be absolutely unbearable and still is in certain circumstances." -Alex

When you become developmentally delayed for whatever reason, our primitive reflexes that naturally should have stopped working by age three continue. This can wreak havoc on the brain and cause underdevelopment. This has NOTHING to do with intelligence!!! Here are many examples of what can happen. Let us start with the vestibular system which is very important in how a child behaves and learns. When the vestibular system is underdeveloped the child will compensate by engaging in movement such as spinning, rocking, or jumping to help their brain pay attention. This is why many teachers see children rocking in their chairs daily. As teachers we find this annoying and we will often admonish the child and ask them to put the legs of the chair back down. I have definitely been guilty of this in the past. There are also kids whose vestibular system is overdeveloped. These kids will do everything to avoid movement. A classic example of this is a child who will not sign up for many sports, ride roller coasters, or hang upside down.

When the midbrain is underdeveloped you may see children create their own white noise by screaming, humming, or talking to themselves. These kids also love bear hugs. We use to call my youngest daughter love bug because she was always asking for hugs. She was listening to her body and was giving it what it needed.

Changing activity is nearly impossible for them and hair brushing may become a battle. Also the brain may not give the signal that the stomach is full. These kids can also become stuck on a simple thought. Change can be really hard with these kids.

What happens when the proprioception in the central nervous system is underdeveloped? What does proprioception mean? Proprioception refers to how your body moves through space. Some of the behavior that is common when you cannot feel a body part is tapping your foot, chewing, and rocking in your chair and then falling out of it. Can you believe the chair can feel slippery to a child with a compromised proprioceptive system? When this system is not working it is hard to tell how much pressure you use to hold your pencil. These children will either hold it too loose or too tight. They will often erase their paper too hard causing it to rip. These are the kids that will pet the dog too hard or play too roughly with other kids. These children can also be seen touching the wall as they navigate the halls going to their class. The concept of personal space eludes these kids.

A child's brain can also be underdeveloped in the speech and language centers. If you are in survival mode all the time it is hard to talk. If the cortex of the brain is needed to help keep the body upright and balanced it does not have time to do its own job of developing language. It takes a lot of concentration to think and then say what you are thinking. It is actually harder to talk than to walk.[10]

---

[10]"Brainhighways" Web 16 Mar. 2016

There is also an unknown 6th sense that most people are not familiar with called interoception. This sense is very important to a developed brain because it relates to all the sensations we feel in our body. This includes pain, temperature, itching, heart rate, hunger, thirst, breathlessness, stretch and pain from the gut, tickle, nausea, sleepiness, sexual desire, sensual touch, movements of digestion, posture, blushing, swallowing, gagging, vomiting, and the feeling one gets when they have to go to the bathroom. Thinking about not having any of these sensations would be a real loss to any child and keep them out of sync.

Chapter 6
DOCTOR/HEALERS WHO ARE THEY?

Now your perfectly healthy child has a vaccine injury and/or is getting sick all the time. What now? The sicknesses in my daughter came in different forms. My oldest daughter had the chronic ear infections. My middle had a two month bout of colic. My youngest developed temporary asthma with developmental delays unbeknownst to me. So if allopathic medicine is no longer an option for you unless you are in an accident where can you go?

Chiropractor

Let us talk about the amazing doctor/healers out there. We will start with the chiropractors who, interestingly enough, knew before anyone else the dangers of vaccinations and they were called the quacks. If I could rewind in time I would have taken my oldest daughter to a chiropractor. Why would you keep having your daughter treated by the same practitioner if the diagnosis is ongoing? I have asked myself that many times..... there clearly is a problem that the pediatrician does not have an understanding of because after the vaccine injury occurs you are referred out. For example chiropractors know that if you adjust the upper cervical region of the body, muscle relaxation can occur which allows the ears to drain naturally. Imagine that!

Which chiropractor do you go to? My advice would be either a Maximized Living, Elevation Health, or Network Chiropractor. If you prefer gentle touches like I do and an emphasis on breathing a Network Chiropractor would be your choice. I have had experience with all three and the knowledge that they can give you as well as how they work with your body is life changing. At the time it was a bit difficult to get my youngest daughter to lie down on the table. Her body would be all stiff and tense. She did not want to lay her head down. Fight or flight was definitely at play. There was one time when I took my daughter to her appointment and she refused to get out of the car. I was at my wits end and I walked in without her. I had heard that there was a behavior center that I could take her too. I had the address written down and kept it in my purse. So I spoke to the chiropractor and told her what I wanted to do. She told me if you do that they will just drug her. Wow! That stopped me dead in my tracks but I was still feeling very desperate. Thankfully the doctor went to my car and we were able to coax my daughter inside for her much needed treatment. This is where I learned we have neurotransmitters in our stomach and I began to get an understanding of the gut brain connection that is so present in "Autism". I also was able to call her at the drop of a hat and bring my daughter in when things were getting out of control. She was a blessing in my life back then. I know the moms reading this can definitely relate. There are angels are out there, we just have to find them. Sometime later I went back to her because I was in a car accident and part of my treatment was my first much needed massage and detox experience with the infrared sauna and the ionic foot cleanse. Goodbye brain fog and hello morning person! We are fearfully and wonderfully made when we get our natural energy flow back!!!

Even though I saw this doctor to treat my daughter I will never forget the wisdom in the form of a book called ""Fight For Your Health: Exposing the FDA'S Betrayal of America" that I bought from this chiropractor at her urging. The knowledge I gained from this book gave me more time with my ailing father. I will go into this in detail in my next chapter.

Structural Energetic Therapist

If you are an "Autism" mom or dad and you are on your child's long journey of recovery you can very well, because of the stress involved, find your own health deteriorating. I was no exception to this. In fact it is not uncommon to suffer from symptoms similar to the soldiers who have come from the battlefield. I am referring to Post Traumatic Stress Disorder (PTSD). Many "Autism" moms and dads are in a constant state of fight or flight. We are always on alert for the next meltdown. Our conversations with our child are guarded.

I became overweight, could only go down the stairs one step at a time because of the pain. I also contracted a two month bout of bronchitis and got a hiatal hernia. I could no longer bend down or sideways because of severe stomach spasms. Off to the computer I went to begin my research. It is my belief the internet has saved so many lives. Doctors do not like Dr. Google. Just a tip, I always Google, Dogpile, or Bing natural treatment for –fill in the blank. The healing advice out in our universe is in great abundance!

Have you ever heard of a Structural Energetic Therapist? I never did either but I found one in my town and after a couple of sessions was able to improve my hiatal hernia 90%! "This is a full therapy which addresses structural pain and builds physical performance to its highest levels." I will be honest I found this experience to be somewhat painful but given that I was already in pain what did I have to lose? I find this healing modality fascinating the way it allows the body to heal itself. This practitioner can help with structural imbalances and core distortion. The techniques they use include Kinesiology (study of human movement), muscle testing, postural analysis, cranial/structural techniques, directed myofascial (muscular pain) unwinding, emotional energy release, acupressure (meridians), scar tissue and adhesion (abnormal membrane surfaces) release, deep tissue therapy and other therapeutic bodywork techniques. [11]

Naturopath

Another healer that I have used in my journey is a naturopath. What is a naturopath? This specialist uses a form of alternative medicine that includes homeopathy, herbalism, acupuncture, diet, and lifestyle counseling. As a side note, because of my daughters extreme anxiety issues blood draws were not even on the table for us. We scheduled this at a hospital one time and my husband and I could not physically get her out of the house. I love how these vaccines poison your child's blood to the point where you no longer can get their blood tested. WOW! Where else do you go but outside the box? All my daughter was required to do here was to put her hand on a cradle and have her energy, signals, and stressors of the body

---

[11]"Structural Energetic Therapy." Web 02 Mar. 2016

assessed. This bio-energetic medicine has been in Germany for over 80 years! "The body stressors include chemicals, heavy metals, viruses, bacteria, parasites, fungi, possible food allergies or catastrophic emotional events." The goal is to return the body to its natural energy state. This next three sentences are very important especially when it comes to "Autism" "A healthy body can handle a small amount of these "interferences". However, if you are sick, low in energy, always catching colds, or you have skin breakouts, rashes, pain anywhere in the body, depression, sleeping problems, weight gain......this indicates that the stressors in your body are interfering with your ability to lead a normal life. If this state continues for a long time, disease will set in, or you might already have a disease." [12]

    I find this very concerning for the vaccine injured population in light of Dr. Bradstreet's suspicion of undetected cancer that I talked about in the previous chapter. A word of caution with this kind of practitioner; I would tell the naturopath that you would like to address one problem at a time and not have your child or yourself become so overwhelmed that the treatment remains incomplete. Many of our children are so sensitive to taste that the form in which they take their treatment needs to be a very important consideration, the younger the child the easier to treat. Do not put this healing off! Do the work!

---

[12] 'holisticoptionsinc." Web 02 Mar. 2016

Holistic Pediatrician

You probably have noticed I am a little bit anti-pediatrician in light of what has happened to my children and so many more as I write this book. Vaccine injury is NOT RARE. In my town I have had the fortune of having a pediatrician/author who became a Holistic pediatrician. He saw what was happening in his practice and he also had his own personal health challenge where he found himself having to go outside the box and seek integrative medicine so he could heal. This is the doctor I went to when I found out how toxic my daughter was and then he referred me on to a Defeat Autism Now doctor which is now called MAPS (The Medical Academy of Pediatric Special Needs). He will remain my daughter's doctor until she is 21. This doctor has gone to the Concierge's model where you pay a monthly fee and the insurance picks up most of the remainder. I have the comfort of knowing I have access to a holistic pediatrician who emphasizes extensive nutrition, vitamins, and herbs. He also has an understanding of the immune system and what part the gut plays. The emotion piece which may be the most important piece is also addressed. Parenting support is also part of this model of care. This is a wonderful model of care but I would again work with the doctor and not treat everything at one time. Treating a vaccine induced brain injury can be very overwhelming. If you keep the treatment as simple as you can and build on it you will have more of a chance of recovery. It is my hope that more allopathic pediatricians will wake up and realize what they have been participating in and turn their practice into full support both physically, mentally, and emotionally for these "Autism" families and return these children back to greatness.

There are some other healers on my list that I have not had the opportunity to visit yet. I will briefly explain their healing modalities.

Cranial Sacral Therapist

This practitioner practices a soft touch noninvasive form of bodywork that works with the bones of the head, spinal column, and sacrum. We know the heavy metals in the vaccines can change bone structure. The objective of this treatment is to let go of compressed areas to get rid of stress and pain. I am reminded of a visit to the pediatrician when my middle daughter, in high school, all of a sudden was told she had mild scoliosis. Yep, it just appeared out of the blue. Interestingly, her cousin of the same age also had a more severe form of scoliosis which required her to wear a brace for a year, just coincidence!

Homeopath

Homeopaths treat with the belief that the body has the ability to heal itself. This healing practice also came from Germany starting in the late 1700's. There are two types of homeopathy. They are Classical and Heilkunst. Classical Homeopathy selectively treats what the living being cannot handle. Heilkunst practices sequential homeopathy which means remedies are prepared to treat everything that has happened over a lifetime simultaneously. Homeopathy is very safe to use for every age including with our four legged friends. The remedies used in both types of homeopathy are made from natural sources (ie. minerals and plants). Classical Homeopathy is more affordable than Heilkunst because it uses one remedy at a time. They are both FDA regulated! The reason for this is because Classical Homeopathy was practiced long before allopathic medicine, the health model practiced in the mainstream today.

Emotional Release Practitioner

I believe this practitioner is very important in treating any disease condition or life event that is emotionally devastating. All of us have heard stories of people dying of a broken heart. This is a body mind technique which allows not just mechanical or body memories to be let go, but significant emotional components as well. Remember hiding negative emotions in our cells lowers our frequency.

Acupuncturist

This practitioner stimulates acupuncture points with needles to clear blockages so energy flow can be brought back into balance.

Integrative Medicine Specialist

This doctor/healer treats one cell at a time. The treatment includes IV-therapies, supplements, nutrition, and other natural treatments. Integrative medicine puts the patient at the center addresses not only the physical, but the emotional, mental, social, spiritual, and environmental influence. The critical missing piece in allopathic medicine is the failure to address the whole body since everything in the body is connected.

The Melt Method

The practitioner who practices this method includes a treatment that can bring you pain free living, a balanced nervous system, and healthy connective tissue. meltmethod.com

I know there are many more different kinds of healers out there. I am learning about more and more as time goes on. I hope I have enlightened you to a little as to what is out there. I feel like we are just beginning to learn how our wonderfully designed body REALLY operates and heals itself. These are very exciting times!

Now on to my Dad's story.......

Chapter 7
MY LOVING DAD 1921 -2013

His Life

My Dad was born on March 9, 1921 in Eindhoven, Holland. He was the second youngest in a family of 7 brothers and sisters. His dad worked and his mom stayed home and raised the family. I do not recall many details on my Dad as a child. I know at one time he took up boxing much to his family's dismay. A wonderful sport for the brain because of the movements involved that cross the midline of the body. I also recall he struggled academically in school which caused a teacher to move him to a business track. He has a memory of seeing houses blow up across the street during World War II. He also was summoned to join the German army. My Dad was very smart though and during his physical they took his temperature and left the room. While they were gone my father engaged in some calisthenics to get his heart rate up before the next testing. When they saw how high is heart rate was he was deemed ineligible to join the German army!

Before the war my Dad had met my Mom and they had a long 7 year engagement in large part because of the war. They married in 1948. My father during this time worked for Post Telephone and Telegraph. My Mom became pregnant with what she thought were twins but turned out to be a 10 lb son. Because of the baby's size he was in the birth canal too long and subsequently died shortly after his home birth. It was a very devastating time for my parents. By this time a couple of my Dad's brothers had left to live in the US and the war was over but the effects of it were far from over. The young couple was feeling very vulnerable and wanted to live somewhere safer. Also having just lost their first son they were looking for a change and my Dad liked the pictures coming from America!

In 1952 the young couple said goodbye to their families and country, got on the boat and immigrated to America. The boat docked in Chicago and my Dad's brother and their sponsor were waiting for them. They soon found an apartment. My father began working at Zenith where his brother also worked. My mother found a job at Sunbeam. I think this adventure was harder on my Mom then my Dad and my Mom who was very homesick found herself returning back home for a visit. While living in Chicago they were active in the Dutch Immigrant Society, so it was here that they found family again. Four years from the time they set foot on American soil I was born and their family began. Two years later my sister was born and then they moved to a house in the suburbs. My youngest sister was born three years later and now their family was complete.

By this time my father decided to attend night school and get his Engineering Degree in addition to working his full time job. I really admire this about my Dad. What a sacrifice they both made! I remember so often wanting to go see my Dad on the weekends but I knew when the bedroom door was closed that meant he was studying and no one could bother him. This went on until I was in 4th grade. He went to night school for 10 years!!! It was such a relief when he finished his Mechanical Engineering Degree from the Illinois Institute of Technology. The time had come where we could see Dad more and do more things together as a family. My Mom and Dad would now be able to socialize the whole weekend! My parent's social life involved partying with their Dutch friends who became our surrogate aunts and uncles. My early childhood memories included joining Girl Scouts where my Mom was a leader, attending Catholic school and then public school, ballet lessons, and being bullied in 7th grade. My sisters were also in Scouts and took piano. We were allowed one activity besides Scouts. We frequented the rummage sales at church and spent many vacations renting a cabin in Wisconsin. We also spent our summers in Holland about every 5 years to visit family. In 1969 my Dad got a promotion and we moved to Huntsville, AL. That was a shock especially for my Mom who had gone to a French Boarding School in her early years. She considered Alabama Hicksville. It was perfect timing for me considering the bullying I was encountering in Junior High School.

I found you could not meet more friendlier and hospitable people than in Alabama. No one is a stranger there. I found it very pleasant and no more bullying. My Dad settled in his job and started playing piano again. Our house was now big enough to have one and he had more time to enjoy his hobby. I loved hearing my father play. He would go on to join the church choir and play for them for many years until his health began to decline.

As I am writing this I have very little recollection of sickness in my family growing up. My sisters and I all had the rite of passage of the chicken pox, measles, and mumps. My middle sister did get rheumatic fever and we all had to be shuttled to our Dutch aunt and uncle's house for a few days until she recovered. I had the odd ear infection here and there. In elementary school my Mom's knee gave out as she was doing a lunging exercise with Jack LaLane in front of the TV. She had to go to the hospital for surgery. When I was in high school my Mom had found a lump in her breast but thankfully it was benign. She also had a blood clot from taking birth control pills and was ordered to bed for a few days. I never recall my parents taking daily medication for anything as I was growing up.

My Dad went through a depression around the time I graduated from college because promises at work had not been kept. It was a difficult time. We know now depression is also very much a medical condition that involves what is going on inside the body. It would be interesting to know if he had been treated with drugs during that time.

Heart Disease, Low Fat Diet, and Statins

It was in the late 80's when things started going wrong, starting with my Dad's heart. Dad's sister and his mother both died young because of heart conditions. I am not convinced this is a hereditary condition as mainstream medicine parrots. Stress also most likely played a role. Things were not easy at his job. I think it is also related to diet. Our diet at that time was a typical American diet of meat, starch, vegetables and desert. My father loved making a delicious liquor coffee too. He also loved making sugar with butter on a slice of bread. He did have kind of a sweet tooth. My parents being Dutch enjoyed their cup of tea always accompanied with a baked good.

In 1989 my father underwent a triple bypass. He was then put on a low fat diet and later prescribed a statin drug which we now know is very dangerous to the heart, the brain, and the immune system. All the talk back then was about the importance of keeping your cholesterol low. His doctors totally ignored the Framingham study which began in 1948. This study involved 5,209 people between the ages of 30 and 62 who were divided into two groups. One group ate little cholesterol and saturated fat and the other group ate larger amounts. Every 5 years comparisons of the two groups were done. We now know data from this study revealed that you can eat as much or as little cholesterol, animal fat, or saturated fats as you like and it will have no effect on your blood cholesterol levels. [13]

Retirement Community

In 2005 my parents decided to sell their house and move to a retirement village in town. It was time to downsize and live simpler. My Dad's walking and balance difficulties were not improving. They moved into a 2 bedroom apartment with a patio. They would be able to eat in the dining room every night if they so chose. If only the food was healthy which it was not. This became more of a concern for me as things got worse for my Dad. The interior of the building where they lived was decorated to the hilt and resembled a very fancy hotel. If only the beautiful decor would have mimicked the wellness treatment he so desperately needed.

In 2007 I had been referred to the chiropractor that I talked about in my previous chapter who told me to buy the book "Fight For Your

---

[13] Tennant, Jerry, MD Healing Is Voltage: The Handbook Third Edition United States: Publisher Not Identified, 2010. Print

Health: Exposing the FDA's Betrayal of America." There was a particular chapter that got my attention called Death by Statin. Because of my experience with the disaster of psychotropic medication with my youngest daughter I was already not a fan of medication. I learned in this chapter, a study called Mr. Fit, the largest dietary study of cholesterol lowering in men, showed a correlation between the lowest cholesterol and highest rates of cancer. In particular there was a lawsuit involving Lipitor which was the exact statin my Dad was on. Pfizer, the maker of Lipitor pushed this statin on people who had never had a heart attack as well as people who have had a heart attack. My father was in the first category. It was only intended for people who had suffered a heart attack. The most alarming side effects were losing muscle, interfering with energy production, and compromising the immune system in the body. At the time my Dad was struggling with his balance and we did not know why. He may have even already begun walking with a cane. After reading this chapter I called my Dad, Mom and my 2 sisters and they agreed we need to talk to his "doctor" about it. Much to my surprise the "doctor" did not fight us to keep him on it.

Cerebellar Ataxia

My Dad was now walking with a walker and around 2008 he was diagnosed by a neurologist with Cerebellar Ataxia. My Mom told me the neurologist would not tell my Dad for a whole year what was happening to him. It took my Dad's family practitioner to have a conversation with the neurologist and convince him to tell my Dad the truth about what was happening. Of course the neurologist had no answers and the family practitioner was the one who had given him all his mercury laden flu shots all these years, the irony of it all. When I first heard of this diagnosis I was in disbelief. I had actually never heard of this diagnosis before. To be honest I was so wrapped up in my daughter's "Autism" there was no room on my plate to thoroughly research another diagnosis.

I made the observation the diagnosis of Cerebellar Ataxia has a lot in common with the diagnosis of Guillain-Barre Syndrome. I was somewhat familiar with this side effect because at the time my middle daughter was entering college and the school wanted to give her the meningitis vaccine which has this same side effect. Given my middle daughters negative effects to vaccines I was able to obtain an exemption. The Guillain-Barre Syndrome is described as follows "varying degrees of weakness or tingling sensations in the legs. Muscles begin to lose their ability to respond to the brain's commands, commands that must be carried out through the network. Wow! This sounds so very similar to what happened to my Dad and this was a known side effect of the flu vaccine. In fact upon further investigation according to the National Vaccine Information Center's website "adult influenza vaccine injury claims are now the leading claim submitted to the Federal Vaccine Injury Compensation Program." I decided to do further follow up on the hrsa.gov website to take a look at these claims and see if I could see some similarity to my father's diagnosis. Unfortunately this information is not available. The website says "it has been moved, removed or temporarily taken off-line."

Since there was no "cure" things got progressively worse. I do remember one day while visiting at my sister's I spent a whole day researching all the 7 medications my Dad was on at the time and the side effects which were not pretty. I also had a conversation with a local compounding pharmacist in my parent's area who went over the side effects with me. One of the medications destroyed the mitochondria which is not that unusual when it comes to many medications I have since learned. I was very familiar with the importance of the mitochondria having sat on the Autism Mitochondrial Task Force out of Boston since its inception. Many children on the Autism spectrum have a mitochondrial dysfunction and my daughter exhibited many of the traits. When you are not a "doctor" you have no influence and it would be another full 6 months before my Dad would agree to start getting off some medication and on to supplements. Whenever I would suggest it he would just smile and shake his head, maybe laugh a bit. He was programmed like so many of us are to "trust your doctor" My sisters were also involved in the "health" field and going outside the box was very foreign to them. Because of his health condition continuing to go south a decision was made to move him to assisted living. In this facility it meant my Mom would now be about a 5 minute walk from my Dad in the same building. We actually had to negotiate that my Mom would be allowed to visit my Dad without having to come in from the outside to the front entrance of assisted living. Thankfully the administration complied. Unfortunately my Mom and Dad would no longer be allowed to have their meals together. The food in assisted living was also abysmal for these chronically ill people and the physical therapy offered was the bare minimum. Occupational and breathing therapy did not exist. If you are in assisted living you have difficulty getting around and traveling for more therapy becomes difficult. Their inactivity just puts them farther into their diseased state.

It did not take long before my Dad went into a wheelchair and moved to skilled nursing. He no longer had the strength to stand up on his own. Soon we would see him begin to struggle with his speech. I found myself talking to my sister about the same technology I saw at the Autism conferences I had attended to help the kids who were not talking to communicate. As time went on I was learning more about cerebellar ataxia and during one of my many independent research sessions on the computer I learned that electromagnetic pulse therapy could help with this diagnosis. So I went in search of this technology in my parent's hometown. There was one Chinese medicine doctor who had this technology and I was able to secure an appointment for my Dad with the family on board. Now to pull this off was a really big ordeal. We had to have a van take my Dad to the doctor's office while he was in his wheelchair. This appointment had to be made in advance and the days they transport had to coincide with the office hours of the doctor. They also had a limit as to how many miles they would travel. Thankfully we were able to make this work. It is stunning that the allopathic model requires very sick people to make their way to the doctor's office. This really needs to change. It is time for the healthy doctor to start making house calls.

It was a bit precarious to get my Dad's wheelchair into the doctor's office because the office was under construction but thanks to the van driver we were able to get my Dad there. The only thing I did not realize was that the examination table was not adjustable and the doctor did not have the staff to lift my Dad on the table to do the electro magnetic pulse therapy. When the nurse saw the problem she started crying. I was really surprised that this doctor did not have the support staff to help my Dad. Do people who are in my Dad's condition never see him? I still do not know the answer to that question.

We were given a wonderful supplement and I saw a difference in my father's strength! He could not lift his foot onto his foot stool before and now he could! My Dad even made an attempt to stand up with the help of the railing but he was not able to do that. I went home thinking maybe I should hire some body builders and make another appointment. As time went by every time I talked to my Mom about it she was just getting more and more overwhelmed by the whole situation. I kept playing the game what if in my mind. I knew the food he was getting was abysmal. I bought my Mom a blender so we could make my Dad some protein shakes at least while I was visiting. I was also becoming more aware of the florescent lighting in his room and how that was affecting his already low cell frequency. But that bordered on crazy talk with my family.

I had also learned about the healing effects of living ionized alkaline water and made sure my Dad and Mom were drinking as close to that every day. They were not convinced to buy an ionizer but I did find a health food store where my Mom could pick up alkaline water at the very least. I knew acidity plays a huge role in chronic illness. There was one time where I stayed for two weeks and hooked up my ionizer to my Mom's kitchen faucet. When I walked into my Dad's room he was slumped over in his wheelchair because he was in pain in his back. I went back to my Mom's room and drew some very high alkaline water (11.5ph) and used cloth napkins and dipped them in the water. I knew this water opens up the pores from the skin. I applied the cloth napkin to where my Dad was experiencing his pain and 20 minutes later the pain was gone and he started playing his keyboard. I also noticed how blue and swollen his feet were so I gave his feet a bath in the living water and the pink color came back as I rubbed them. It was fascinating to watch! We are fearfully and wonderfully made!!!

My dream was to have everyone have access to this living water in this retirement community but the Director there had no interest in learning about it. Yea I guess it would put a cramp in his system there. Everyone would stay in independent living and live longer!!!

Last Days

I made my last visit to see my Dad in January 2013. At the time I had no idea it would be my last time. I was coming up to meet with the "team" and see what other healing modalities we could apply. When I got there I was told my Dad was not feeling well and was in bed. The meeting with the team preceded and ideas were discussed and it looked like things were moving in the right direction. The resident doctor never made an appearance at this team meeting. I was there visiting my Dad in the evening and I was talking to the nurse who I had become close with and who knew my Dad well. She started crying and attempted to show me what my Dad's notes said and revealed to me that the doctor made the decision that it was my Dad's time to go. I was in complete shock and did not understand why this was kept for our family at the "team meeting" where the "doctor" did not even bother to show up for. At the time they were also giving him Ensure which is full of processed cancerous sugar and should not even be given to a healthy person let alone a very sick person. My father was having more trouble breathing and I bought him a personalized steam inhaler and a healthy substitute for Ensure. I was not ready to give up but I could tell everyone else seemed to be. I felt like I was living in the twilight zone. People came in from "hospice" expecting us to embrace their services which my Mom thankfully declined. We can have our own hospice after all we were in a skilled nursing setting! I found out that the resident doctor owned the hospice too. What a racket! I was trying my best to wrap my head around what was happening and realized now I would be staying for a funeral. It was just a matter of time now. The head of nursing decided a few days before my Dad would leave this planet that he should eat a peanut butter and jelly sandwich. Seriously? I guess she had to check that box off. I also had the experience of the cleaning crew coming into my Dad's room who was at his death bed and clean his room with their toxic cleaning supplies. I could barely breathe upon entering. Things were gradually going from bad to worse in my mind. I let that cleaning guy know these cleaning methods were very inappropriate and harmful to anyone let alone very sick people. He apologized. I am sure he had no voice in the cleaning supplies chosen.

So the morphine was ordered and it was now a matter of time. There is no greater pain than having to watch someone you love die like this and I know many of you reading this have been there. No one should die like this. Just like how positive our body responds when we eat food from its natural source we should allow our body to die naturally. This is not natural. I think if our body does not become ravaged by toxins over a long period of time we can die a natural death. Dying when we can still walk on our own should be our goal.

Before my Dad died I was able to play music which he loved. I found myself playing the song "Wild Horses" over and over. I could not watch him die. It was too painful. My friends on Facebook were a great source of support. They had gone through it before. They knew what to say. I stayed out of the room on that last day. I did go in after he died. I had to see him that way so I believed it happened. He looked so white. I knew he was no longer there. My passion to change why people are sick and die grew even stronger.

Chapter 8
PERSONAL DEVELOPMENT

What is stopping you from growing your own mind? There is a difference between taking knowledge in and developing and empowering the mind you already have. Did we ever entertain this idea in our formal education? I know I never did. I never recall having the opportunity to take a personal development class. I will have to admit I was pretty low in the mind growth department all my life until I joined a network marketing company. Can you grow your mind without network marketing? Absolutely!!!

With more kids on the spectrum today than ever before the subject of personal development becomes even more crucial to give these kids a sense of self-worth. They have to feel good about something and see inside themselves in a positive way is a great place to start.

When I saw my youngest daughter suffering both physically and mentally and no doctor had answers it was time to find some. This was a no brainer for me. This was a time when I went back to reading many books, something I had very rarely done since college. Yes really! Did you know that the more you read your thirst for knowledge comes back? You just want to know more and more. Fortunately the topics I was studying, ADHD and Autism were just evolving and there was so much to learn and think about. I was once again taking in knowledge.

But once you attain some knowledge what do you do with it? This is where personal development can play a role in how you are perceived when you share it with others. You have to talk to people in a way where they know without a doubt you believe what you say.

So let us break down what the words personal development mean. According to audioenglish.org personal used as an adjective means affecting particular person or his or her private life and personality. Development means the ongoing process that something is growing and getting better. Have you ever thought of the concept of having thoughts that come to you be able to empower you? Now in order for you to do that you have to be very positive. You also have to have the belief and confidence in yourself.

Self-Talk

How do you do that? One of the ways to do this is by practicing self-talk. When you understand that words have frequency and this affects our cells you start to grasp how powerful this can be for you. An example comes to mind. I had taken some time off from substitute teaching to write this book. One day while I was getting ready to start my day of writing the phone rang like it normally does in the morning. It was a school asking if I could teach that day. I said "no I am taking some time off to write a book." I hear the lady on the line say "Oh I have tried to write a book I hope you don't get writer's block" I thought to myself did she really just say this? I assured her I would not and quickly hung up the phone. But just that thought in my head was freaking me out. So I just started saying aloud I will not get writer's block......I will not get writer's block.......over and over. So by doing that exercise I was able to overcome the negative thought this conversation put in my mind and I did not get writer's block!

Affirmations are another way to practice self-talk. Just commit to saying a statement every morning after you get out of bed that you can feel empowered by. An example will be "Today I will find purpose in my life." Now when you say it say it with meaning behind it and at a volume to match. As you say it your mind is listening. So throughout the day you will be thinking it and you will constantly be reminded as you engage in other activities of whether this particular activity is related to your purpose in life. Say it more throughout the day if you want to. Say it like you believe it. Exude confidence!

The Power of Fear

There is nothing to fear but fear itself. We have all heard that before. How do we define fear? According to Psychology Today fear is an emotional response induced by a perceived threat, which causes a change in brain and organ function, as well as in behavior. We see this when our hands get clammy, our heart starts beating faster, or we feel those butterflies in our stomach.

How does fear play into personal development? Well here is an example. I would not even be an upcoming author if I would have feared the unknown. A few years back I saw an ad while I was scrolling through my feed on Facebook about a coaching seminar in my town. I really had no idea what I was getting into but the word coaching intrigued me so I thought I would give it a try. I had heard a lot of successful people have coaches. All I was giving up was one Saturday.

There was no cost involved. What did I have to lose? If I would have let fear creep in to my decision making I would not have gone. I did not know anyone else that was going. In fact until I got in the room I was thinking it had to do with real estate. It turned out it was all about personal development which I was hearing on my company calls every day. Some of it I had heard before but you really cannot hear too much of this. Every time you hear it it becomes more ingrained in your unconscious mind.

I was also chosen for the mastermind. I was so excited! What is a mastermind you ask? A mastermind is a group of people who come together for support and encouragement. We were each given an opportunity to talk about what our purpose in life was and where we were headed. The entrepreneur/mentor who ran the company came to the mastermind and guided us in our vision. I left very excited!!! Just attending this one day event which I knew nothing about has led to so many more opportunities with more on the way.

Fear keeps us from moving forward. Fear is right where our opponents want us. Fear paralyzes us. There are also positive aspects of fear when we face it and overcome it. An example is engaging in a physical activity that on the face of it you deem it impossible to accomplish. Like minded people in a group can help you overcome your fear of participating in an activity you could never see yourself engaging in. When you push through your fear the sky is the limit. This is how you apply mind over body. Overcoming your obstacle in life will take precedence over physical pain.

Get Uncomfortable

Let us talk about the subject of being uncomfortable. I think in order to grow personally this is a requirement. I have learned this first hand as an advocate for my daughter in the schools and exposing allopathic medicine for many years. You are automatically made to feel uncomfortable when you are questioning the status quo. But that is actually when you need to keep going in your belief and in your truth. Looking at how the word uncomfortable is defined we see the prefix un which means not and comfortable meaning affording comfort.

I was very comfortable or so I thought before I knew that my children had been harmed. We had the basics including a comfortable home, food, and clothes. I was involved in PTA, volunteer activities, Mother's Day Out, and carpooling. We enjoyed movies, shopping, watching TV, getting together with friends, traveling and living abroad. My husband's job was secure. What more could I ask for? I was comfortable.

This all started changing very gradually when my youngest daughter was in 7th grade and I learned the truth behind the ADHD/PDD-NOS, cognitive and behavior struggles, and violent meltdowns. How do you remain comfortable once you know the truth? Does not the humanity in you want to shout it to the world so this does not happen to more children? There was a very eerie silence. You were the crazy one. Were you the only one that was seeing this? Whenever you broached the subject you would get the deer in the headlights look. You spent hours alone researching on pub med trying to make sense of everything you were hearing. You were constantly looking for a school that would fit your out of sync child's needs. You were going from doctor to doctor. Your family did not see what you saw. It is not easy living in an uncomfortable state for a long time but if you persevere you will begin to see the fruits of your labor.

When I look at how far I have come in knowledge, my ability to help people in my community and how my online community is still teaching me every day, my state of being uncomfortable far outweighs the alternative. I have grown far more as a person than I would have had I remained comfortable and kept my mouth shut. The things that use to be important to me no longer are. The meaning of being rich is not about how much money you have it is about your mindset. Is everybody on board yet? No but we have made a lot of progress and there are now many more people who have woken up. The deer in the headlight look is long gone. Now there is only resignation. Babies are being saved and drugs and medical procedures are now being questioned. Alternative medicine is being considered. The truth is being told!

I will close this topic by encouraging everyone to challenge yourself, to never stop learning, to overcome your fear of being different, to find that confidence that is in you and embrace it. Never fear the truth. The truth will set you free.

Mind Growth Events

Since I have been around thought leaders for the last couple of years I have noticed a pattern; many of them became broke before they became successful. They found a way to invest in themselves. They made it happen. So as a result of this observation I believe there is good debt and bad debt. I believe investing in yourself is good debt. Sometimes it comes down to having faith when investing in a personal development program.

Now if you live where I live in a vacation capital the opportunity is abundant and free when it comes to personal development. The two coaching companies that I have had the pleasure of learning from are the JT Foxx organization and the Peaks Organization. With the JT Foxx organization I have attended Mega Partnering, Mega Marketing, Mega Speaker, and Family Reunion. I also received an invitation to attend the Millionaire Mind Intensive which led to a Reignite event. Thanks to JT Foxx I attended Guerilla Business School which is associated with the same company Peaks Potential, which is part of Millionaire Mind Intensive. From there I met James McNeill of the Guru Builder where I learned the importance of writing a book as a guru. I have attended free events and paid events and they have both enriched my mind and gave me the confidence to move forward in life. Everyone I have listed speak all over the globe!!! The connections you make at these events are invaluable. There is something very powerful when you are in the company of like minded people. When you leave these events you are no longer alone in your journey and support is in abundance online, in a local club, and weekly teleconference calls. Another empowering growth tool is the

Brainathon by John Assaraf which I found free on social media. It seems like the more you embrace these thought leaders your opportunity for more growth just snowballs. It is very exciting and empowering. I would encourage all of you to take that next step in life and keep your growth momentum going!

One thing I have observed is successful people in life have coaches. A coach helps you see yourself as others see you. A coach holds you accountable. They guide you to the next level. They are not afraid to call you out. They push you farther than you think you can go and then some. They give you a vision. They lead you to your greatness. The money you spend on coaching you will get back tenfold. For people who are struggling financially right now google coaching and mastermind group and you will be lead to Difference Makers who are changing lives for free. I also love Darren Hardy who sends me a motivational text everyday completely free. I cannot tell you how many people there are out there in the universe wanting to help you take your life to the next level. The opportunity for growth is in abundance. We are so blessed with such life giving people who have been blessed and now want to pay it forward.

Credit Card Roulette

I will add that it may be necessary for a little while to play what I call credit card roulette. If you can keep up with your balance and use cards with no interest this may be a way to invest in yourself. I believe this is the best investment you can make. You will only be increasing your personal wealth when you can empower, believe in yourself, and exude the confidence that will attract your clients and customers. The law of attraction is very real! Always be open to listening to the voices around you too.

Read

Another way to develop yourself personally is to pick up a book on personal growth. There are so many books out there waiting to set you on fire. We are so blessed to have so many people who have taken their time to become an author and share their wisdom from the many experiences they have had. Start a book club and hold each other accountable to the goals you set for yourself as a result of your growth learning. Set aside an hour a day to read about personal growth.

Chapter 9
MOTHER'S PAIN and CALL TO ACTION

I could not end this book without sharing some snippets of the real raw pain of autism moms I know including my own from a post on a recent Face book page. Some of these snippets may appear like ramblings and have no structure but I can assure you they have a purpose. The purpose is for you the reader who may or may not have an idea of what it is like to have a child with autism aka vaccine induced brain injury feel the great sense of loss of what could have been that we autism moms experience daily and know intimately all too well.

When I hear my 19 year old daughter talk about having met a boy online on a free dating site and saying she does not want to go out and get hurt again. When my daughter asks me to take her driving in a parking lot when she still has not passed her test for her permit. When we were shopping for her newly painted room yesterday and realizing this is the shopping I should have done with her a year ago as she was getting ready to go to college. When I leave to teach today having to be thankful that my daughter has a friend that will be picking her up so she can work out and maybe has someone to spend her day with. When my daughter nails the singing part of her audition but when it came to the dancing she was cut right away because her brain could not process the steps fast enough. When I shared this post with my husband and all I get is silence.

"As a Mother to hold your recently vaccinated child in your arms as they nurse for hours, seem lifeless, and we are told that is normal. To not have questioned then only years later breaking free from this "standard of care" with scrutiny. When finally reading the history of vaccines, the sinister and sick manipulation of the public literally brought me to my knees in shock, sadness, and despair. I hope my kids will understand that at least I was able to rethink this and save them from any more potential harm. To not have billions of dollars in order to fight such evil forces, I depend on our Creator. Proverbs. "The truth stands the test of time, but lies are quick to be exposed."

"Kimberly transitioning into Kindergarten from the county special ed preschool program. "She's so bright and high functioning, she'll be perfect for inclusion" I was told. This is the Holy Grail right? Yeah, my daughter will be in the mainstream. I was told the other program, a special day class was too low functioning and not at all suited to her needs. I told the special education director I wanted to observe both programs prior to her IEP so I could be an informed participant. Walking into the inclusion program, you might as well have punched me in the stomach and smacked me upside the head with a 2x4. There was no way my daughter could handle the chaos of this room. I envisioned her curled up in a ball under a table for most of the day. They described the program, and I left feeling sick to my stomach, there was no way this program would work for my daughter. I went to the "low functioning"SDC and it was the perfect environment. Mixed grades mixed disabilities with 7 kids and 3 adults. A very calm atmosphere where Kimberley could learn how to go to school.

"Standing at the playground and having other kids approach you to ask "what's wrong with your kid?" Hearing you now 15 year old son say he wished he didn't have autism so his life wouldn't be so hard. When my 15 year old son's speech teacher in 9th grade tells me he isn't pronouncing 3 letters correctly including the "L" that you can't talk around, though 10 years ago his former speech teacher tried to get his IEP dropped because he was "no longer having articulation issues" When his brother's friends are throwing balls really hard at him in PE and he had to stop participating in class to get them to stop hurting him. When he says he was born different and doesn't want to live."

"When my 13 year old daughter gets upset and wants to go live with the homeless people at the beach and starts packing a bag because she thinks they will be her friends. When the only friend she has at school is controlling and manipulating her daily. When she wants to make other friends at school but is not able to initiate speaking to them."

"When my 17 year old wants to go to MIT or Berkley and his test scores are fantastic but he cannot remember to write down his homework because of his executive functioning issues. Ten years of executive functioning goals at school and it's still not being addressed properly."

"The regret of not knowing I could have gotten an exemption. The regret of not knowing what was in the vaccines. The regret of not knowing about the genetic component of MTHFR. The regret of not knowing aluminum is a neurotoxin. The regret of not knowing the importance of autoimmune history in the family. The regret of letting myself be bullied into getting a flu shot during my pregnancy."

"My son told me with tears running down his face that the principal, assistant principal and some teachers were giving away treats and letting kids tape the principal to the wall.......but only the kids that scored 75%or higher on some practice tests. The rest of the kids not only could not participate but did not get their name called out in the cafeteria in front of all the other kids. My son told me he feels like giving up because he tried his best but feels like he will never be good enough!"

"My pain is watching my 23 year old son experience self-injurious behavior and not be able to figure out the cause. Also, as I age I have deep seated pain, as to his future, as providers I have met are uncaring, untrained, and uneducated in autism. It's very heartbreaking. All the first in life we missed out on cause pain daily."

CALL TO ACTION

1. Schedule a screening of the documentary VAXXED in your hometown. All information can be found here. vaxxedthemovie.com
2. Call your Congressman and ask that Dr. William Thompson be subpoenaed so the investigation of the fraud at the CDC can begin.
3. Ask Congress to repeal the 1986 National Childhood Vaccine Injury Act and hold manufacturers liable for injury caused by their vaccines.

4. Demand that the single measles, mumps, and rubella vaccines be made available immediately.
5. Make sure all vaccines be classified as pharmaceutical drugs and tested accordingly.
6. Have business size cards to hand out with the vaccine ingredients on them. These can be obtained for free by calling 800-939-8227 or emailing VIC@vacinfo.org with your mailing address.
7. Let your car be your voice! A car decal kit can be purchased at vaccineliberationarmy.com
8. Let your friends and family know that immunizations are NOT REQUIRED for school. This is a STATE MANDATE and exemptions can be obtained in most states. Contact NVIC.org for state specific information. Leave your child home when obtaining your exemption.
9. Take advantage of Public Access Television Programming to get the word out.
10. Hold screenings for the movies "Bought" and "Trace Amounts" at your local church or community center.
11. Attend a rally at the CDC. They will be announced on the Thinking Moms Revolution Facebook Page
12. Make a donation for someone you know with Autism to Teamtmr which is the 501C3 for the Thinking Moms Revolution. Our website is teamtmr.org
13. Design a T-shirt with a message that speaks to you and that will spark a conversation.
14. Join NVIC.org so you can keep up to date on what medical freedom issues are occurring in your state. This organization was co-founded in 1982 by Barbara Loe Fisher, whose child was harmed by the DPT. Thirty four years later this organization is the

beacon of our movement with Barbara at the helm. She personally called me when I posted my story on social media in 2008 to tell me it was because of the vaccines which I had already concluded.
15. Check out the Autism meet up groups and attend one of their meetings for a future speaking opportunity to further educate.
16. There is also a website called learntherisk.org which is a call to action for everyone who wants to educate. Here you can find downloads available to hand out about vaccine ingredients, chemicals are chemicals, doses, and say no. Also there are information cards and bumper stickers available for all topics concerning the wellness movement. Join the Facebook page called Learn the Risk too!
17. Join tacanow.org   Talk About Curing Autism. Find a Chapter near you or start your own.

My intention in writing this book was to help you avoid what has happened to me and my family. I would like to see you not have any empty chairs around your dining table during the holidays. I also hope I have empowered you to seek your greatness, take control of your health and live a life of wellness. This story will continue because I believe we are in the middle of a very big paradigm shift. By the time this book comes out there will be even more information out there to help us reach our greatness. The universe is waiting for you.

I will end this book by telling you a story I heard about how lobsters grow. The texture of a lobster is very soft and jelly like. This very soft lobster lives in a hard shell. As the lobster grows he becomes very uncomfortable because there is no give in a hard shell. The only way he can continue to grow is to go under a rock, shed his shell and make a new one. In comparison to a patient who gets drugs from his doctor and remains comfortable as long as he stays on the drugs. If a lobster would go to a doctor he would never grow! The moral of this story is adversity is the motivation for growth. Embrace your greatness, get uncomfortable, and growth will be in abundance!

Mark 10:43: Whoever wants to be great must become a servant

ACKNOWLEDGEMENTS

I wish to personally thank the following people in the order of my journey for their contributions of knowledge, inspiration, and other help in creating this book.

God- Whose voice spoke to me clearly and whose presence is always guiding me.

My loving husband Jim who supported me financially and took over in our home so I could focus.

My beautiful daughters Meghan, Jenny, and Maria who let me be that strong Mom.

My college roommate Nan who was open to journeying toward wellness with me.

My late mother-in-law Ginnie who was my rock during my darkest days of "Autism"

My students in my class who are my best teachers.

Doctor/Healers who were my teachers: Dr. Joseph Cannizzaro, Dr. David Berger, Dr. Corrine Allen, Dr. Paul Rousseau, Dr. Don Colbert, Dr. M.K. Murphy, Dr. Domminick D'Anna, Dr. Stephan Sinatra, Dr. Tim

McKnight, Dr. Peggy Parker, Mojka Renaud LN, A.P. , Dr. Jerry Tennant, Dr. Dan Yachter and Dr. Bate

My cheerleader, warrior Mom, and Co-Author Laurie

My business mentor Jason whose encouragement has helped me believe in myself.

The Thinking Moms Revolution who share my passion and journey. My personal development mentors- Rich, Sam, Nicholas, Brooke, Jim, Lee, Darren, and John.

JT Foxx and his organization -You helped me grow in ways I did not know were possible.

Melanie - You helped me through my biggest networking adversity so I could move forward.

Lee - Inviting me to my first Peak Potentials event that continued strengthening my mindset.

Healers - I always had to have pen and paper handy whenever we talked.....Beth, Gail, and Zoey

James MacNeil - The Guru Builder who made my experience of vibration real.

Raymond - My publisher who surprised me by inviting me to his amazing book camp.

Nu_design - My book cover designer who captured my vision.

Naval-My book architect , and website designer, who believed in my work and kept me challenged.

Lisa- My editor

ABOUT THE AUTHOR

Mary Pulles Cavanaugh is a Mom of three beautiful daughters. She holds a Bachelors Degree in Social Welfare from the University of Alabama. She also has a background in medical assisting. Mary became an avid independent researcher in 2007 by necessity when her youngest daughter was diagnosed on the Autism spectrum aka vaccine induced brain injury at age 11. This led Mary to a greater awareness of the sick care system that is so prevalent today. Her eyes were opened even more when her late father was diagnosed with cerebellar ataxia and the similarities she saw with "Autism".

In 2014 an amazing door opened for Mary to join The Thinking Moms Revolution and become a co-author of the book "Evolution of a Revolution: From Hope to Healing How Thinking Parents Are Recovering Their Children and Uncovering the Truth". She has also recently submitted a 2nd Chapter for another book by The Thinking Moms on Puberty and Autism.

What keeps Mary going on this very exciting journey is the knowledge that we are fearfully and wonderfully made and we all have greatness within us. When she is not recovering Autism, telling the truth about vaccines or fighting for medical freedom she may be seen teaching at a local middle school and unleashing the greatness of the tweens. Mary can be found on facebook, linked in, twitter @max4metals and thebookongreatness.com.

Resources Which Continue To Enhance My Journey

Detox   amajordifference.com
                 max4metals.mycoseva.com

Special Ed Law   wrightslaw.com

Genetics   23andme.com
                 medomics.com

Books

Backyard Secret Exposed by Beth Sturdivant
backyardsecretexposed.com

Cure Tooth Decay Heal and Prevent Cavities with Nutrition by Ramiel Nagel

Earthing by Clinton Ober, Stephen T. Sinatra, MD and Martin Zucker

Fight For Your Health: Exposing the FDA'S Betrayal of America

Excitotoxins by Russell L. Blaylock, MD

Healing Is Voltage Third Edition by Dr. Jerry Tennant

A Shot in the Dark: Why the P in the DPT Vaccination May Be Hazardous to Your Child's Health by Harris L. Coulter and Barbara Loe Fisher

Brain Training brainhighways.com lifekinetikusa.com

Vaccine Injury - vaers.hhs.gov

medalarts.org - search engine for vaers database to look up specific reactions or vaccines

Living Water Hq0 Ionizer-   max4metals.myqsciences.com
　　　　　　　　　　　　　　　checkouthq0.com

Mind Growth Events

millionaireunderdog.com
millionairemindexperience.com
thegurubuilder.com

Personal Development Leaders

richvosler.com
darrendaily.com
myneurogym.com

Circulatory and Vascular System   avacen.com

Appendix – References

Journal Articles

Evidence of Toxicity, Oxidative Stress, Neuronal Insult in Autism.
Journal of Toxicology and Environmental Health, B Crit Rev, 2006 Nov/Dec; 9(6)485-99

Hepatitis B Vaccine and the Risk of CNS Inflammatory Demyelination in Childhood.
Neurology 2009 Jun 9, 72(23): 2053
Braillion, A.; Dubois G.

A Comprehensive Review of Mercury Provoked Autism.
Indian Journal of Medical Research 2008 Oct; 128(4): 383-411
Geier, D.A.; King, P.G.; Sykes, L.K.; Geier, M.R.

Thimerosal Neurotoxicity is Associated with Glutathione Depletion: Protection with Glutathione Precursors.
Neurotoxicology 2005 Jan
James, S. Jill PhD (University of Arkansas)

Autism: A Brain Disorder, or a Disorder that Affects the Brain.
Clinical Neuropsychology (2005) 2, 6, 354-379
Herbert, Martha R.

Poor Cognitive Development and Abdominal Pain: Wilson's Disease.
Scandinavian Journal of Gastroenterology 2006 Mar; 41(3): 361-4

Oxidative Stress in Autism.
Pathophysiology 2006
Chauhan, Abha; Chauhan, Ved

Website

"Autism & Vaccination Quotes", http://www.whale.to/vaccine/quotes1.html, accessed on 4 Dec 2009. Copy included with letter.

The Book on Greatness

Printed in Great Britain
by Amazon